Theo's presence in the [...] catch her breath. She [...] how handsome he was, or the way [...] body reacted to the smell of his aftershave.

He looked up in surprise at Addy. "What are you doing here?"

She raised her eyebrows. "You mean you aren't part of the plot to destroy me?"

He sagged down into a seat with a look of bewilderment.

"I've not been here long enough to plot anything," he said easily. "And I'm not important enough, and I don't have enough hours in the day. But—" he took a breath and looked amused "—I might be up to plotting some kind of coup at a later date."

She leaned forward. "And why would that be?"

He sat back and folded his arms. "Let's just say I'm watching and waiting. Biding my time."

"Are you planning on becoming leader of the world?"

He shook his head and grinned at her. "You forget I have a three-year-old. Leader of the world is tame. He'd expect me to be leader of the universe."

NURSE'S DUBAI TEMPTATION

SCARLET WILSON

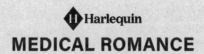

MEDICAL ROMANCE

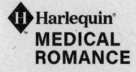

Harlequin®
MEDICAL ROMANCE

Recycling programs
for this product may
not exist in your area.

ISBN-13: 978-1-335-94299-9

Nurse's Dubai Temptation

Harlequin Enterprises ULC
22 Adelaide St. West, 41st Floor
Toronto, Ontario M5H 4E3, Canada
www.Harlequin.com

Printed in U.S.A.

Scarlet Wilson wrote her first story at age eight and has never stopped. She's worked in the health service for more than thirty years, having trained as a nurse and a health visitor. Scarlet now works in public health and lives on the West Coast of Scotland with her fiancé and their two sons. Writing medical romances and contemporary romances is a dream come true for her.

Visit the Author Profile page
at Harlequin.com for more titles.

To any family that finds yourself missing a key part,
I see you and I hear you. Love is everything.
Treasure your memories.

Praise for
Scarlet Wilson

"Charming and oh so passionate, *Cinderella and the Surgeon* was everything I love about Harlequin Medicals. Author Scarlet Wilson created a flowing story rich with flawed but likable characters and…will be sure to delight readers and have them sighing happily with that sweet ending."

—*Harlequin Junkie*

**Scarlet Wilson won the 2017 RoNA Rose Award
for her book
*Christmas in the Boss's Castle.***

PROLOGUE

Lyon, France

THE HOSPITAL ADMINISTRATOR looked at him again. 'Dr Dubois, do you understand what I'm telling you?'

Theo was never normally lost for words. But suddenly the leather chair he was sitting in felt alien to him, the bumps on his skin like some tropical disease, and the muddled thoughts in his head were surely some kind of pre-seizure thing.

Thing. That was where his medical brain had gone. Because absolutely none of this was normal. It wasn't real. It was a dream. Or a nightmare.

He felt something touch his hand. Colette, the hospital administrator, had moved closer and nodded to the gendarme in the room. Colette was formidable. A woman in her early sixties, she was always dressed impeccably and ruled this hospital with her iron will alone. No one crossed her path and lived to tell the tale. But today she was being nice to him. He recognised the look of empathy on her face, and it broke him just a little. She repeated her previous move and nodded to the gendarme.

But Theo wasn't ready for the gendarme to speak again.

'I spoke to her on Wednesday,' Theo said. 'I'd seen them a few weeks ago and offered to help again. I asked if she wanted me to go and get Max. She didn't sound great, but she told me she was fine. She told me she didn't want my help.' His voice drifted off.

The gendarme cleared his throat. 'Fleur—Ms Bernard was found on Friday after neighbours alerted us to the sound of a crying child. It seems as though it was an accidental overdose. We found some papers in her home that indicated you were her next of kin, and she wanted you to look after Max.' He paused for a moment. 'I'm assuming you're Max's father.'

The words jolted Theo back into this new reality. 'What? No. Fleur was my girlfriend at school. We haven't been together for more than ten years. But she asked me to be Max's godfather, and I agreed. She'd had a falling out with her family...' he took a deep breath '...because of the drugs.'

He raised his head as the enormity of the situation started to take hold. 'What does this mean?'

The gendarme looked a little awkward. 'Social

services will be in touch with you about custody of Max. Do you happen to know if Ms Bernard has a will?'

Theo gave a wry laugh as he ran his hands through his hair in pure frustration. 'Yes, I know,' he said. 'I got her in touch with a free will service when her habit got worse. Told her she had to be responsible for Max. She wasn't listening to anyone, wouldn't accept any help. Social services had put support in place for her, but,' he sat back in the chair, his voice getting smaller, 'Fleur didn't want help. Her addiction had well and truly taken hold.'

A chill settled on his skin. He'd never admitted those words about his friend to anyone. She'd been on a path to destruction. The last time he'd seen her in person, she'd slammed the door on him. He'd been relieved when she'd answered the phone on Wednesday. He thought things might be getting better.

A hand rested on his shoulder. 'I'll take some more details from you, and social services will be in touch—probably tomorrow,' said the gendarme.

Theo nodded automatically. He spent the next ten minutes handing over Fleur's parents' details, the company who'd done Fleur's will, and asked everything he could about how he could arrange the funeral, and collect Max's things.

By the time the gendarme left, he felt as if he'd run a marathon.

He took a few moments, just breathing, and finally held up his hands to Colette. 'What am I going to do?'

Colette sat down in the chair next to him. 'Let me help you, Theo. Won't Fleur's parents organise the funeral?'

He shook his head. 'Fleur was a late baby. They're both in a care home now. Her father has dementia.'

Colette nodded. 'What about you? How equipped are you to look after a baby? Do you have family that can help? A partner?'

He shook his head again. 'My *papa* has multiple sclerosis, and my *maman* is his full-time carer.' He gave a smile. 'And no partner. Currently single.'

A furrow creased his brow, as the first wave of panic hit. 'I hardly know anything about kids. I've looked after Max lots of times, but I just winged it. I don't actually know how to do this for real. And what about my shifts? How on earth will I get childcare to cover my shifts?'

Colette lifted a piece of paper from her desk. 'First thing, ' she said, 'don't panic. Take a breath.' She was watching him carefully. 'And, even though your friend may have put it in her will, if you don't think taking care of Max is the right thing to do, you need to have that conversation with social services. They won't ask you to take him unless you're fully prepared for all that entails.'

His stomach clenched. Was this what he would have chosen? No. Was this how he thought his life might go? Not really. But when he'd agreed to be Max's godfather, he'd known this could happen. When he'd lost his temper and told Fleur she had a responsibility to her child—to think about his welfare and make a will—he'd known who she would name. He had no idea who Max's father was. Fleur had never told him. Whoever the guy was, he hadn't been in their lives.

Theo took a deep breath. 'I'll take him. I want to take him. I'll make things work. I have to.'

She turned the piece of paper around and showed it to him. 'I wouldn't normally do this. You're a great cardiologist. We're delighted to have you here. But I understand how difficult things can be. I just got this. They're looking for specialist doctors. A cardiologist like yourself would be in high demand. They're offering very attractive packages for the right candidates. If you tell them you have a child and need childcare arrangements, I'm sure they'll be able to help.'

'Dubai?' Theo was speechless. He'd never considered working anywhere but France, his home. Sure, a lot of his friends were working in places all over the world, but his brain had just never gone there.

Colette gave a nod. 'Tax free too. Think how much you could save. Work there for a few years, come back with plenty in the bank, and it'll help your future with Max.'

All of a sudden, his brain started to go places. He currently had a small flat, and a mortgage. Long-term he'd need something bigger for him and Max. If he could save enough for a big deposit, he might even be able to drop his hours further down the line, to make sure he could meet all Max's needs.

Colette smiled. 'Just so you know—even those of us who carried a baby for months, and pushed him out—we all winged it. None of us know what we're doing. Even the ones that read the manual.'

He sighed, his shoulders finally relaxing for the first time since he'd been called into this office. Colette continued. 'I won't pretend that being a one-parent family isn't tough. It is. I know. But you can do this, Theo. I have faith in you. So, let me just say, I'll help you out over the next few weeks. And if you get this job, I'll still be here at the end of the phone for you. Day or night. Things can get on top of you. Sometimes it's overwhelming. But I can't tell you the joy you'll also feel watching a little person grow and thrive. Being a parent is a privilege. You're about to embark on the greatest adventure of your life.'

Her tone of voice was warm. He was seeing a whole new side to the hospital administrator—who was rumoured to know her own nickname of Attila, and not object to it. He reached into his pocket and pulled out his phone, scrolling until he found the last picture he had of Max and him together. Max was three, with rumpled blond hair. His T-shirt was stained with raspberry sauce from the ice cream he'd just eaten, and he was throwing his head back and laughing as Theo held him. The joy that Colette had spoken about was evident.

He took a deep breath and felt something settle over him. This was real. His future had just changed. He could do this. He turned his phone around to share the picture and smiled at Colette. 'Meet Max. He's just about to take over my life.'

CHAPTER ONE

Three months later

ADDISON BATES WAS NUMB. She'd been numb for the last four months. Ever since her fiancé had cleared out their joint bank account and disappeared into thin air.

Since then, it had been like peeling back the layers of an onion to find just how much debt he'd accrued in her name, and just how illegal some of his activities had been. The last straw had been the extra mortgage, in her name, on her property.

She'd considered herself a good judge of character. Sensible with money, and with her heart. But Stuart King had ruined all that. She'd left her engagement ring behind when she'd packed up the house, since she knew now it couldn't possibly be real.

The heat hit her as soon as she stepped off the plane in Dubai. It was a dry, searing heat. Not one she was used to. But she would have to get used it.

It was her only possible chance of getting out of the escalating debt she now had against her name.

Of course she'd involved the police. But they'd politely told her the fraud investigation could take more than a year, and in the meantime her credit rating was lower than the belly of a snake and would likely remain that way, even if it was proved that Stuart had taken out the debts in her name.

So, Dubai it was. She'd known a few people that worked here. Her role as a sister in the coronary care unit back home, with previous experience in Cardiac ITU, made her a good candidate at the many specialist hospitals throughout the area. Her salary was more than she was used to, and came with an apartment in an apparently nice area.

She also wanted to get away from the mutual friends she'd shared with Stuart. She'd been aware of the judgemental looks and the apparent distrust from people. Did they really think she was in on it?

She shuddered. Dubai was a new start for her. At least she hoped it was.

The apartment was in a closed complex—the building was an actual skyscraper. There was a concierge. It was reassuring. She had to show proof of identity before she was allowed in and given her passkey. She was also given a list of rules and told that her belongings had already been delivered.

The floor-to-ceiling glass windows in her main living area gave a view over the wonderful landscape of Dubai, with all its majestic sights. She pressed one hand to the glass. It was like a city of clouds up here.

As she pulled her hand back, she could see her hand print and she shuddered. This whole place was pristine. She was already making a mess.

She'd asked for furnished accommodation and this looked like a show home. Sure, the apartment only had one bedroom, but the white walls and pale furniture gave the place a sense of space. That, and the views. The only room that didn't have a view was her bathroom, and she was thankful for that. Her bedroom looked out over the city too, and she wondered how it would feel to sleep here at night, practically up among the stars. The kitchen was small but practical. There were laundry facilities, and the whole complex had a swimming pool and gym area too.

As Addy looked around, she couldn't help but shiver. This place was lovely—perfectly respectable for her needs. But the rooms seemed to echo around her. The canvas was blank, and she'd thought that she wanted this, but now that she was here?

She took a breath and sank down into the comfortable cream sofa. It was overwhelming. Her interviews online, her resignation at her previous post, the way she'd stored up her few possessions before her flat was taken from her. The flight to Dubai almost seemed as if it had passed in the blink of an eye.

Now she was actually here, to do a job. In a country where she couldn't speak the official language. Though English was widely spoken here too. The hospital who'd employed her had reassured that she would likely work mainly with European patients.

But the thought of reporting there tomorrow suddenly seemed too real.

Addison sighed and looked around. She was lucky. Of course she was. She had a chance to earn good money, recover financially, then decide what she wanted to do with her life. It was nobody's fault but her own that she'd ended up in this position. She was too trusting. Too amenable. Or, at least, she had been.

That Addison Bates was gone.

The Addison Bates who was going to be the new sister in the cardiac ward, in the world-renowned Spira Hospital in Dubai, would be none of those things.

She wasn't here to be everyone's friend. She wasn't here to accommodate all the other staff.

She was here to give the best possible care to

her patients, to make sure their cardiac care or surgeries were successful, their recoveries uneventful, and the staff worked diligently under her.

It was time to adopt a whole new mindset.

And she was ready.

CHAPTER TWO

'DR DUBOIS? Mr Koch needs his pain meds reviewed.'

Theo took the chart from nurse and had a quick check of the notes. 'No problem, I'll go and review him, then prescribe something more effective.'

He was settling in. The hospital was vast. and while he'd thought his former workplace in Lyon had state-of-the-art equipment, it was nothing compared to what Spira Hospital had underneath its roof.

Nothing was too expensive, equipment was replaced frequently, and the staffing levels were above any he'd experienced before. Each nurse only had two or three patients to look after. He was supervising only one ward area, and another few beds in coronary care ICU. He had Theatre time every day in the specialist cardiac theatre, and didn't need to fight amongst other surgeons for time.

The on-call rota was less than he was used to, and he and Max were gradually finding their feet.

It had been like jumping into a freezing cold pool of water. Unprepared, and out of his depth. Max knew him, but had only stayed on a few occasions, and Theo's place hadn't been child friendly to begin with. Moving from France to Dubai had only been delayed by waiting for Max's passport to arrive. There had been no problem with Theo becoming responsible for Max, and that had him both a little sad and angry. Max was initially shy, but fun and intelligent. The world should be fighting for this kid—but Theo was the only one standing.

As for Spira Hospital? It was every bit as good as the frequent TV adverts showed it to be. His apartment was lovely and comfortable. The childcare arrangements better than he could have even imagined. And the area they lived in had lots of facilities.

Except it was lonely. There hadn't been a chance to make friends yet. His colleagues were courteous and kind, but it wasn't the same as having a wide circle of friends that you could phone at a moment's notice, or knock on their door to have a beer and a bit of company.

Theo gave a final glance at his computer, mentally listing the other things he needed to do this morning, and stood up to go and assess Mr Koch.

He'd barely taken two steps when the unmistakable noise of an emergency buzzer sounded. It was dull, not directly in their area, but everyone went into autopilot. They'd been warned earlier that the arrest paging system was being reconfigured today. Although he wasn't on call, there'd been no confirmation the system was working correctly again. He turned to the room down the corridor where the buzzer was sounding and started to run. It was through the double doors. He could see an unfamiliar colleague up ahead grab the emergency trolley and tug it towards the room.

He knew this wasn't one of his own patients. He had four other cardiology colleagues who had patients in this hospital. But his body was designed to always respond to the sound of an emergency buzzer—no matter where he was.

As he crashed through the doors, he grabbed the back end of the trolley, giving it a helpful push into the room.

The woman pulling it let out a yelp. 'Careful!' She scowled, her eyes flashing. He'd never seen her before, but she was wearing burgundy scrubs, the sign of a charge nurse.

'Who's the patient?' he asked, ducking around the trolley and moving to the head of the bed to assess the situation.

'No idea,' was her short response. She glanced

up at the monitor. 'Ventricular tachy,' she said, before pressing a button to inflate a blood pressure cuff already on the patient's arm.

There was a nursing assistant opposite, dressed in grey. He was tugging the pillows out from under the patient's head, and pulling them so they were flat on the bed.

'Someone tell me something,' said Theo, trying to keep his tone light, even though the situation was clearly serious.

'I called the code,' said the nursing assistant. 'One minute she was talking to me, the next her eyes just rolled and everything started alarming.'

Another nurse ran in, glancing in surprise at the people in the room. 'This is Isabel Aurelis,' she said quickly. 'Twenty-one. Multiple episodes of fainting and fast heart rate. We're investigating for Wolff-Parkinson White but she literally just got here. She's just had her bloods done. Hasn't even had an ECG yet.'

'Surely she had one pre-admission?' snapped the charge nurse. She had an unusual accent. Her dark hair was caught up in some kind of clasp, her expression was serious.

'And who are you?' asked the nurse. Theo could hear the hostility in the air. There was no time for this.

The other woman had stepped to the bed and was currently feeling for a carotid pulse at the side of the neck. 'I'll be your new charge nurse,' she answered. He placed her accent—Scottish, and strong. It would be easy to lose track of what she was saying. Her gaze flicked to Theo. 'No pulse.'

Theo moved fast, taking in the information displayed on the monitor and lifting the paddles from the defibrillator. 'Pulseless VT,' he said out loud. 'I'm going to shock at two hundred joules.'

He waited while the nurse placed the thick gel pads on the patient's chest area. 'Where is Isabel's doctor?'

'Dr Gemmill is due in sometime in the next hour. He knows Isabel is arriving.'

'Page him.' Theo glanced around. 'All clear.' He wondered how Dr Gemmill would feel about him taking over the care of his patient. It didn't matter—this was an emergency situation. Some doctors could be odd about another consultant stepping in. Once he was sure no one was touching the patient, or the bed, he delivered a shock, watching Isabel's back give a short arch as it was delivered.

His eyes went to the screen and he noticed the charge nurse's fingers went to Isabel's carotid pulse again. 'A flicker,' she said in a low voice.

Inexperience and anxiousness could sometimes make individuals too impatient with cardiac events. But Theo knew better. 'Let's wait,' he said calmly. He saw the smallest nod from the charge nurse, who kept her fingers lightly at the side of Isabel's throat.

His eyes went back to the monitor. There was the tiniest blip. After a few seconds, another. And then, finally, the comfort of seeing a QRS complex alongside a normal rate.

He stepped back, and breathed. Just like everyone else in the room.

Isabel Aurelis was a fortunate young woman. If this situation had happened anywhere else—somewhere that a defibrillator wasn't immediately available—it was unlikely she would have survived.

Theo reached for the electronic chart and automatically started adding tests. 'I want a twelve-lead ECG, twenty-four-hour monitoring to make sure we don't miss any future runs, a cardiac echo and I'll prescribe some amiodarone meantime to try and stop any abnormal rhythms.'

'Do you have authority to do that?' the charge nurse asked, a line across her brow.

Theo looked at her again. There was a weird vibe. An off vibe. But he didn't even know this person, and couldn't remember seeing her around here before. He opened his mouth to answer, but she'd turned to the nurse who'd run into the room once the code had been called, peering at the woman's badge for a few moments.

'Layla, you don't ever bring a patient onto this ward without consulting me first. And you certainly don't bring a cardiac patient up here without the most basic tests. No ECG? Has she had any pre-admission tests done? A full history?'

Layla's dark eyes widened. She opened her mouth to object, but the charge nurse raised her hand. 'This is my ward now. This incident will not be repeated.'

It was only a few words, but an icy chill flooded through the room. In any other circumstance, Theo might have raised his eyebrows in amusement. This wasn't how he conducted himself with other members of staff. Looked like this charge nurse was on a mission.

It was almost like she read his mind as her eyes suddenly met his. What an unusual colour. And he felt himself inwardly cringe that had been his first thought. What was that colour? Violet—or a funny shade of blue? Whatever it was, those eyes had a laser focus.

'Addison Bates,' she said in a clipped voice. 'I'm the new charge nurse for this ward. And you are?'

It was the tone of her words. Slightly confrontational, with an edge of challenge. Or maybe it was just the accent and he was misreading things. Whatever it was, it instantly set all the cells in his body on full alert.

'Theo Dubois.' He nodded towards the door, giving her a clear sign to take this outside. He started walking, quickly checking on Isabel's readings and giving a nod to the nursing assistant to remain in place.

Annoyance flooded Addison's face as she followed him out. Once they were clear of the door, he turned to face her. 'I'm one of the cardiologists from the ward next door. I was warned the arrest system was being reconfigured this morning, which was why I responded. So, yes and no. I do have authority to request those tests, though I'm not Isabel's doctor.' He glanced down at the chart. 'Dr Gemmill might overrule me once he gets here, but, until he arrives, I have a responsibility for Isabel's care. And—' he took a breath, aware that he didn't normally act like this, but the new girl had kind of annoyed him '—we don't have those kinds of conversations in front of patients here.' He looked at her badge. 'Charge Nurse Bates.'

He could see instantly she was aggrieved. Her dark pupils flashed and tiny pink spots appeared on her cheeks. He was trying to remember who she reminded him of. It was someone old-school. Someone either his *maman* or *papa* had liked, but the name escaped him right now. He was also trying not to notice how entirely attractive she was. Theo couldn't remember the last time he'd been attracted to someone in his workplace. Considering he'd only been here three months, and now had Max to look after, it wasn't as if a relationship could even be on the cards.

'You're new here. You should take some time to get used to the system and processes in place.'

Sparks practically flew from her. 'It might be my first day, but this is my ward, and there's no way I'm going to have a repeat of what just happened. An unknown patient…' she put her hand to her chest '…coming to *my* ward, with no proper notes, history or tests?'

Theo cringed. He knew what she was saying. He would never work like that, but he didn't want to speak for the consultants on Nurse Bates's ward. Was it wrong that he also liked how feisty she was, and that it totally matched her Scottish accent?

He pushed the thought from his head. 'We have a mixture of patients coming up here, both private and local.'

'I'm well aware of that,' she shot back. 'But the local patients present at Accident and Emergency. They're seen and assessed before they come to us.'

He gave the barest shrug of his shoulders. 'Then you'll have to speak to your own consultants about their arrangements for admission.

They might not agree with having to run all their private admissions through you first.'

She held her hand out towards Isabel's room. 'Well, if this is anything to go by, the current process isn't safe, and I won't stand for it. Patients deserve better.'

The edges of his lips almost tilted upwards. He had to absolutely tell them not to. Because he was quite sure she wouldn't like it. A few strands of dark hair had worked themselves free of her clasp. With the flush currently in her cheeks, and her unusually coloured eyes, the new charge nurse was actually quite beautiful, and clearly passionate about her role.

He handed over the electronic tablet where he'd signed off all his instructions. 'Nice to meet you, Charge Nurse Bates,' he said. 'I've left everything for Isabel recorded. If you need me, I'll be just next door.'

He started down the corridor, then heard her clear her throat behind him. He glanced back as his hand reached the door.

'Addy,' she said. 'My name's Addy.'

He gave her a little nod of his head. 'Theo,' he replied, before disappearing through the door.

How to have a disaster on her first day—Addison Bates was clearly winning at this one.

Maybe she should actually be happy that Theo

wasn't a doctor on her ward. This whole situation wasn't something she would want to repeat, for both professional and personal reasons.

She cringed at Theo's retreating back and turned back to deal with Isabel. Trust her to fall out with the first consultant that she met here, and it certainly didn't help matters that he was probably the most handsome man she'd seen in her life.

Not that she would ever trust a man again. That part of her life was well and truly over. She was here to get a new life, do a good job and work her way out of a financial black hole.

It also wasn't the first impression she'd wanted to make on her fellow nursing staff members. She'd need to resolve that issue too.

Isabel was propped up comfortably in bed now, with the nursing assistant fussing around her, chatting easily, getting her a drink of water, offering to find out when she'd be allowed something to eat. Addy tried her best to paint a smile on her face.

'Isabel, how are you feeling?'

The girl blinked and looked at her, putting a hand to her chest. 'Like I've been hit by a truck.'

Addy smiled at the nursing assistant. 'I'm sorry. I'm Addison Bates, the new charge nurse. I didn't catch your name?'

'Omar.' He smiled. He was around twenty

years older than Addy, and looked like he might have done this job for a while.

'Omar, would you mind finding Layla again, and asking her to chase up the tests that Dr Dubois ordered? And let us know when they might be arranged? Could you also ask her to page Dr Gemmill again, please?'

Omar nodded and disappeared out of the room.

Addy sat down next to Isabel. 'You've had a quite a day,' she said quietly. 'Would you like me to talk you through it and explain what happens next?'

Isabel gave an anxious nod. 'Can I have a bubble tea while you explain?' she asked.

Addy shook her head. 'Not right now, but maybe later. I'll ask you to stick to water right now, until your tests are complete and Dr Gemmill has reviewed them. He might want to take you for some treatment today.'

Isabel gave a sigh and rested back against the pillows as Addy talked her through the event. She explained how her heart rate had increased so much that it was no longer pumping her blood around her body the way it should. She took her time to talk about electrical impulses, and how an electric shock brought everything back to normal—that it was a known type of treatment for this kind of event.

Isabel still had one hand on her chest. 'I don't

want that again. How can you stop this happening to me?'

There was a noise behind her, and Layla escorted in some staff who were wheeling equipment into the room. Layla introduced them. 'Paulo is going to do the cardiac echo and ECG, and Mariam here will take some further blood samples that were requested.'

Addy gave Isabel's hand a squeeze. 'Don't worry, I'll be back soon to explain the rest.'

She followed Layla outside and back to the nursing station. 'Sorry, for the abrupt arrival,' she said. 'We haven't had a chance to be properly introduced.'

Layla gave her a cautious glance. 'I'm Layla, I trained here and I've worked in cardiology for five years.' She gave a nod towards the double doors behind them. 'I go between both wards, depending on the staffing.'

Addy was still feeling on edge, knowing things had got off to a bad start. She hated that, particularly when she was working in a new place and really wanted people to like her. But she had to be true to herself.

She took a breath and gestured for Layla to sit down next to her at the nurses' station. 'I'm sorry about our initial introduction. I can promise you I'm not normally like that. I'm sorry if I upset or offended you by being so direct. I'm obviously new here, and saw some things that caused me concern.' She took another breath. 'Do you mind if I ask you a few questions about the ward?'

Layla gave a cautious nod.

'What happened today with Isabel's admission—is that normal practice here?'

Layla pulled a face and looked a bit uncomfortable. 'Yes. And no.'

Addy frowned. 'So, what does that mean?'

'It means that some consultants do it, and others don't.' She bit her bottom lip. 'Some of the consultants are very casual. They'll either see a patient privately, or take a phone referral and just arrange for them to come in. Although the doctor has assessed them, the patient notes don't normally get sent to us until the patient is actually in the bed. And, if they've seen one of those consultants privately, although they need a string of tests, they don't get ordered until the patient arrives.'

Addy wondered how best to deal with this. She knew for sure there was no way to let it continue. She decided to take a soft approach. 'Layla, you don't know me. I'm Addison Bates, I've been a general nurse for twelve years. I've worked in Accident and Emergency, Cardiology, Cardiac Intensive Care, and assisted in Theatre for cardiac procedures. I've been a ward sister for four years, and like to think I have a problem-solving approach.' She looked into Layla's dark eyes. 'Can you see any issues with the current arrangements we have?'

Layla gave a nod and a sigh. 'I hate not knowing the patient's history before they get here. Sometimes we have to wait a few hours for the electronic notes to arrive, along with the patient instructions. Often we just get a call from one of the consultants, or their secretaries, to say that a male or female patient is arriving, and they'll be along later. Sometimes they give us a diagnosis, sometimes they don't.'

Addison drew in a breath. 'Has anything like what happened today ever happened before?'

Layla wrinkled her nose. 'Not exactly. Some minor issues maybe. But nothing as bad as today.'

'And is it all the consultants that do this, or only some?'

Layla shook her head. 'Just a few.' She pointed to some names on the board next to them. 'None of the consultants in the ward next door do it. Theo—Dr Dubois—who was just here, he's new too, but he's very specific about any of his private admissions coming in, has a whole plan specified, tests prearranged and a time agreed with the ward staff for admission.'

'Theo is new?'

'Yes, he and his little one just got here from France.'

'He has a kid?'

'Yes, a little boy I think.'

She shouldn't be asking these questions. She knew she shouldn't be asking these questions. But they'd just erupted without any thought. Why was that?

Was it the sexy accent that had come out of his mouth when he'd talked? Or was it his tall build, brown hair and soulful-looking eyes?

Addy gave herself a shake. She had poor taste in men. She had history. Last time she'd got herself in a relationship she'd ended up with a re-possessed house and a multitude of debts. Theo Dubois was likely a charmer. And that was the last thing she needed to be around. Hopefully he had an equally beautiful wife who took up all his time.

This job was important to her. This job was a chance to build some resilience, restock her life, and her goals, and try and reset things for herself. There would barely be any time for friendships, let alone anything else.

The only person she needed to concentrate on in Dubai was herself.

Layla was still sitting next to her. 'Let's have a chat about this later,' said Addy. 'I think I can do something to try and put processes in place to help get things better organised.'

Layla gave a shrug of her shoulders. 'Good

luck,' she said. 'Some of the staff here can be a little old-fashioned.' She straightened her uniform as she stood up. 'I'll go back and deal with Isabel until Dr Gemmill arrives.'

Addy nodded as she picked up a nearby notebook and started writing a few things down. She needed to focus. She would spend the next few days on the ward learning as much as she could.

And then…she would make some suggestions.

CHAPTER THREE

HE WAS TIRED, and definitely a little bit crotchety, as he juggled the shopping, his backpack and a very sleepy Max in his arms.

It was barely six pm. The hours at Spira were everything they'd promised to be, with better staffing levels, good childcare arrangements and less on-call than he'd had back in France. But as he looked at the little head resting on his shoulder, he wondered if he'd made the right decision.

Max had been in the nursery-cum-daycare centre for the last nine hours. The staff there were great. They played alongside the kids, taught them some basic language skills and helped keep them entertained, fed and rested. But Max was always exhausted when they got home.

And as a new dad, Theo didn't even know if that was normal or not. He might text Colette later. She'd been true to her word, and been happy to answer any queries he had. She'd even spoken to him late at night, when he'd been worried about Max crying in his sleep and the nightmares he'd been having. Having a soothing, rational voice at the end of the phone—from someone who'd done this before—was a relief. He could, of course, have called his *maman*, but she had enough stresses of her own without Theo adding to them.

As he reached for the keys in his pocket, his shopping slipped from his hand. The contents spilled on the floor just as the elevator doors pinged along the corridor. He couldn't even look up, his eyes fixated on the tub of chocolate ice cream—Max's favourite—that had tipped open and seemed to be melting on the floor like a mini volcanic eruption.

'Whoops,' came the voice with a hint of amusement. 'Let me help you.'

It was that exact moment when Max chose to open his eyes, see his destroyed ice cream and let out a howl.

Things really couldn't have gone worse. Or maybe he shouldn't have had that thought.

Because in the next second he was staring into a familiar pair of violet-blue eyes. Addison Bates gave a jolt as she recognised him, gathering his undestroyed shopping items from the floor. She had a bag of her own, and after a second's pause, she put all the items in together.

Her dark hair was down today, landing on her shoulders in soft waves. She was dressed casually in jeans, a white T-shirt and a lightweight navy blazer. It was kind of impossible not to notice how good she looked.

Max buried his face into Theo's chest while squirming, leaving him with no hands free to help.

'Thank you,' he said quickly, then gestured to his door. 'I'll get inside in a moment and clean up that floor.'

The ice cream trail had almost reached Addison's shoes. She didn't seem too worried. 'Are your keys in your backpack?' she asked.

He shook his head and tried not to squirm himself. 'In my pocket,' he admitted, still keeping hold of the sobbing Max.

She tucked the shopping bag under one arm, held up both hands and raised her eyebrows. 'Shall I?'

He hesitated for only a second. This was clearly going to be the worst new neighbour meeting in the world. He tipped his right hip towards her. 'Be my guest.'

She didn't fumble or mess around. Addison slipped her slim hand into his pocket. He felt a short wave of heat from her palm through his thin trouser pocket as she scooped out the electronic keys and scanned his door.

Certain cells in his body started a Mexican wave that he was absolutely intent on ignoring.

The door clicked open and he breathed a sigh of relief. 'Thank you,' he said, hoping for an easy retreat.

'I'll stick these in the kitchen,' she said, gesturing to the shopping she'd crammed under one arm and then heading into his apartment.

'Sure,' he murmured, taking the briefest of seconds to wonder how she knew where to go, then realising their apartments were probably very similar.

He walked in, paying attention to Max, stroking his hair and muttering soothing words as they both flopped down on the comfortable sofa.

Max wasn't a child who did big dramas. He was clearly overtired, and Theo hoped it would settle soon. 'My scream,' the little guy sobbed into Theo's neck.

'Don't worry about the ice cream,' he said quietly, 'I'll get some more tomorrow.'

As he kept talking in a low voice to Max, it took him a few moments to realise that Addison had clearly looked around his kitchen, found some supplies and was outside, on her hands and knees, cleaning up the mess from the pristine tiles that lined the hallway.

'You don't have to do that,' he said, feeling embarrassed, but she waved one hand and gave a small shout in return.

'No worries.'

He smiled at the broad accent. Addison Bates had been quite sharp the first time he'd met her, but he sensed there was something more beneath the surface. Everyone had a reason for working in Dubai, everyone had a story. He'd learned that quickly since he got here.

For many it was money. The rate of pay over here was much better, along with the tax benefits. For some, it was the country and the experience. For others it was escaping a past life for whatever reason, and finding a new place to call home. Or it was the work-life balance. Better pay, a possible reduction in hours and the added benefit of childcare.

Even though it had only been three months, Theo knew that, back home in Lyon, he would have struggled to manage. There was still the occasional hiccup here, but nothing that, so far, had been insurmountable.

As Max started to settle in his arms, he continued to watch Addison, cringing as he saw just how gloopy the ice cream was to clean.

Max was paying attention now too. 'No ice cream,' he said in his saddest voice.

Addison's head lifted and she shot Max the biggest smile. 'Actually, I might be able to help.'

Her gaze shifted to Theo, and even from this distance those violet blue eyes were mesmerising—more so when they held his gaze. Was he imagining this? It had been a while since Theo had dated. Maybe he'd just forgotten all the rules. How could a few seconds feel like the longest stretch in the world?

And then she blinked, and returned her attention to the floor she was cleaning.

Theo stood up and set Max down on the floor. 'Here, let me get that,' he said, still embarrassed at their second meeting, walking out to the corridor to join her. Maybe it wasn't only Max that was overtired and he was just overthinking things.

'It's fine,' she said again, moving into his kitchen area to deposit the used cloths in the refuse bin. She picked up the shopping bag she'd left on his countertop. 'And I might be able to save the day.' She tipped out the contents of the bag that had a mixture of his and her groceries.

There, in amongst the fresh fruit and vegetables, cold meat and cereals, was an identical tub of chocolate ice cream. She bent down to Max. 'It seems that you and I have the same favourite ice cream. How about I give you this one, and you can still have some tonight?'

Max's eyes widened. He reached out for the large tub. 'Can I, Theo? Can I?'

He should say no, but he could see the potential joy in Max's face and he didn't want it to be removed. 'That's really kind,' he said to Addison.

'But…' he knelt down next to Max '…we really should share. Would you like to join us?'

There was a moment's awkward silence. His stomach gave a little flip and he realised he might have made her uncomfortable. 'I'm sorry,' he said quickly. 'You likely have a family of your own to get home to.'

He saw her swallow as she met his gaze. 'Nope, it's just me.' She took a breath, 'And I'd love to share some ice cream.' She smiled down at Max. 'And you're really doing me a favour. I was likely going to eat the whole thing myself in front of the TV, so sharing is definitely a better option.'

His brain immediately flooded with a million possible scenarios. She could be waiting for family to join her. She might be the first to get a job here, and other members would come along later. His eyes looked to her left ring finger and he saw it was bare. The one thing that stood out in her words was 'just me'. Then something prickled in his brain. Just how lonely the night ahead she'd planned was.

But how dare he? A night with ice cream in front of the TV was likely what half the population might dream of. He had no business passing judgement.

A small voice broke into his thoughts. 'Do you have spwinkles? We have spwinkles. I can give you some. I have mashmallows too.'

Theo couldn't help but grin broadly.

Addison gave him a curious stare. 'His English is great, but you're French, aren't you?'

Theo nodded. 'His mum was bilingual, and because he was introduced at an early age he seems to have picked it up no problem. The nursery workers at Spira mainly speak English to him and he appears to manage well.' He took a breath. 'Let's get this ice cream out. Why don't you have a seat?'

He gestured towards the table in the main room. Addison and Max sat down together while Theo gathered some crockery and cutlery. He gave the ice cream scoop to Addison as he set out the bowls.

'One or two for Max?' she asked.

'One,' he said, at the same time as Max said, 'Two!'

They all laughed as he gathered the ice cream decorations and brought them to the table. 'Chocolate sprinkles, multi-coloured sprinkles, marshmallows and chocolate sauce.'

He sat down in the chair next to her and gestured to the table. 'And this is why I said one scoop. The sugar explosion after this will be massive.'

Addison smiled in agreement as she scooped out ice cream into the bowls. Max held up both kinds of sprinkles. 'What kind do you want?'

Theo held up his hand for a second. 'Oh, I'm so sorry, I forgot my manners. Max, this is Addison Bates. She works at the hospital with me.'

'Addy,' she corrected quickly. Her eyes met his for the briefest of seconds. 'My friends call me Addy.'

'Addy,' Max repeated as he looked at her. 'What kind?'

She pointed. 'Definitely chocolate.' She pushed her bowl towards him as he shook the tub, giving her a generous sprinkle.

It was clear he liked to be in charge of the sweet treats as he decorated everyone's bowl. 'I'll have to prise them out his hands later,' said Theo under his breath to Addy.

She seemed perfectly at ease sitting at their table, chatting away to Max about nursery and what he liked doing. For a second, Theo felt a sudden chill—what if she asked something about Theo's mum? But maybe she'd heard from elsewhere about his circumstances, because she didn't bring it up at all.

It struck him that he'd never done this before with Max—sat down with another female joining them. He'd spent a few days with his *maman* and *papa* when he'd first taken custody of Max—one for a bit of support, and two because he knew his next stop would be Dubai, and he wasn't sure when they'd all get the chance to be together again. Being with Max on his own had become his new normal, and this right now? It was nice.

'How are you settling in?' he asked.

She pressed her lips together for a second. 'It's certainly different.'

'What do you mean?' That sounded as if she wasn't too sure about her new place of work.

'I mean...' She gestured to the view from his living room. 'The apartments and facilities are nice.' She looked around. 'Mine is a little smaller, but it's better than a million other places I've stayed.' She bit her bottom lip. 'Spira is taking a bit of getting used to.' She reached up and twisted a lock of her dark hair around one finger. At first he wondered if she was nervous, but she looked more thoughtful than anything else.

He gave a contemplative nod. 'For me too. The technology is state of the art compared to what I'm used to at the hospital in Lyon. I thought the equipment we had there was good. But this stuff? Everything has been brand new to me.'

She pulled a little face. 'The equipment has been fine. It's some of the systems and processes that make me flinch.'

He knew immediately what she was referring to. 'You think they're unsafe?'

He watched her as she clearly considered what to say. 'Not deliberately so. But sometimes casual isn't good. I've written some new standard operating procedures for the wards, for all staff, and handed them into the staff governance group for approval.'

'You have?' He gave a half-smile. 'Well, you don't waste any time.'

'I don't,' she agreed, and shifted in her chair.

'So, what brought you to Dubai?' he asked. It didn't seem like too intrusive a question, and he imagined she'd be asked it a number of times over the next few weeks.

'I needed a change,' she said without hesitation. 'I was already a charge nurse in a cardiac unit in Glasgow, and had worked in cardiac ICU and assisted in Theatre for cardiac procedures. My experience meant I had a few jobs to choose from over here.'

'So, you didn't come for the sun, the money and the accommodation?'

She sent him a half-smile. 'Let's just say they weren't my main reasons, but were definitely added extras.'

She gave a little sigh, and he knew better than to pursue that comment. Instead he asked the question that was playing around in his mind. 'Do you have friends over here already—or some that might join you later?'

She shook her head. 'I don't know a single person. And no, no one will be joining me.' She looked down at her nearly empty chocolate bowl as she said those words. There was an edge of melancholy, and he realised he'd accidentally pushed more than he should.

'Well, I'm sure you'll make plenty of friends now you're here. The hospital has good social clubs, its own gym and I think around half of this building is filled with hospital staff.'

'Do you go to any of the clubs?' she asked.

He nodded towards Max, who now had his head leaning on one hand and was stirring his nearly empty bowl. 'It's a bit hard to go to clubs when it's just me and Max. I work enough hours already. I don't want to look for a babysitter to take more time away.'

'It's just you two?'

He gave a nod and hoped she wouldn't ask for any more details in front of Max.

She gave him a thoughtful look. 'Well, if you ever have an emergency, and I'm not working, I'll be happy to help.' She held up her hands. 'Not pretending to be a kid expert, but I've babysat for lots of friends in the past.'

He couldn't help the almost sigh of relief he let out as he gave her a genuine smile. 'That's great, thank you. The hospital nursery and daycare have been my only help for Max, so it would be nice to have an emergency back-up plan. Thank you.'

She shrugged. 'No worries, I'm only two doors down. So just give me a chap if you need to.'

He frowned for a second.

She let out a laugh. 'A chap? It means a knock at the door. One of my many Scottish sayings.'

He smiled. 'Okay, I get it.' He looked over at Max. 'I think it's time for a bath and bed for someone here.' He nodded towards the empty carton of ice cream. 'And thanks for that. I'll replace it, I promise.'

She stood up, clearly taking his words as a cue to leave. 'Don't worry about it. Your boy needed it far more than I did.'

She didn't stand on ceremony. Just gave a wave and saw herself out, gathering up the rest of her shopping and closing the door behind her.

Theo listened to the silence echo around the apartment. Max now had his head on the table and was virtually sleeping.

He hadn't had a female friend in this place since they'd got here. Was Addy even a friend? It was literally only the second conversation that they'd had. But she'd been helpful, good with Max and he'd sensed a certain vulnerability around her.

Maybe that should send red flags to him. Max's mum had been vulnerable. He needed stability for Max. That had to be his priority right now. So, no matter how much he thought she was attractive, and how easy she was to be around, he couldn't let himself get distracted. His relationship with Max had to be paramount right now. Nothing else could interfere.

He inhaled. A hint of her perfume was still in the air around him. His skin prickled. He liked it. And he liked the fact it was still there.

He reached down and picked up Max to take him through to the bathroom. 'Nice lady… I like Addy,' he murmured sleepily as Theo rubbed his head.

'I do too,' Theo responded, feeling a little sad. 'But you're my most important person,' he whispered into Max's ear. 'And we're going to do just fine.'

CHAPTER FOUR

SLEEP HAD EVADED Addy the last few nights. She wasn't sure if it was because of the shift in time zones, or that her thoughts had been invaded by a handsome doctor she was trying not to think about.

But the fact the HR director was waiting to meet her this morning couldn't be good. 'Miss Bates, can we chat please?'

Her stomach did a complete somersault as she nodded and followed her into a nearby office.

The woman gave her a smile. 'Just a small change in some details,' she said hastily.

'What do you mean?' Addy was doing her best not to let panic overwhelm her.

'I've been asked to move you to the ward next door.'

'What? Why?' Addy felt stunned—she hadn't had any time to settle in yet.

The director sent her a sympathetic look. 'We think you might be better suited to the other cardiac ward environment.'

'Excuse me?' What was happening here? Addy shook her head. 'I don't think I understand.'

'It's felt you need some time to settle in.'

'I agree,' said Addy, feeling automatically defensive. 'Which is why I don't understand why you would move me within a few days.' The woman just kept looking at her. Did she think Addy knew more about this? 'Isn't there already a charge nurse in that ward?'

'Yes, there is, we're just going to swap you both.'

'And have they been asked what they think of this?'

The HR director gave a smile. 'You're not contracted for a particular ward—just a particular speciality. And you will both be remaining within that speciality.'

Addy sat back in her chair. 'You're going to have to give me more details. What is this really about? Have I upset someone? Has there been a complaint?'

She couldn't imagine that there had been. All interactions with patients and their families had been good.

Something sparked in her brain. 'Is this because I asked for some processes to be reviewed?'

The look on the director's face told her all she needed to know. It was clear she hadn't wanted to tell Addison herself.

Addy leaned forward. 'What happened on the ward on my first day was unsafe, and could have had a different outcome. Patient safety has to be our first concern.' She used the word 'our' on purpose.

'And it is,' said the director quickly.

'Are you clinical?' asked Addy.

'Excuse me?'

'Do you have a clinical background?'

The director shook her head. 'No.'

'Then how can you really know about patient safety, or how the current processes—or lack of them—put patients at risk?'

Addy put her hand to her chest. 'That's my job. It's my job to make sure our ward is as safe as we can make it. That's why I put those suggestions to the clinical governance group. I'm sorry if some of your consultants didn't like it, but they should at least have the courtesy to tell me.'

'It's been decided you would be better suited to the other ward area. The change will be in place from today onwards.'

Addy straightened in her chair. 'I didn't come here to cause trouble. I came here for a new start. But if I see something that puts my patients at risk, as Charge Nurse, I have a duty of care, and I have to act as their advocate. This won't go away on its own. We *all* have a duty of care to our patients.'

She let the words hang for a few moments before standing up. 'The processes,' she licked her lips, 'I didn't put them forward for one particular ward, I put them forward for the whole speciality.'

The director swallowed and met her gaze. 'I know.'

'And the clinical governance process—it won't be halted once papers have been submitted?' This was really important. One person's ego shouldn't be allowed to compromise patient safety. If it was, she would walk, no matter how much debt she was in.

The director gave her a hint of a smile. 'Once the papers are submitted, they can't be discounted. They'll have to be considered by the whole committee.'

Addy let out a breath. There was still a chance she could make some changes around here.

The director stood up and spoke in a low voice. 'Just move next door, continue to do your job, and keep your head down. The committee processes generally take around six weeks. By that time, you might find that some have warmed to your ideas a little more.'

Addy gave a nod of her head. 'Okay then.'

Her head was spinning. Part of her wanted to have a tantrum. Clearly, at least one of the consultants had thrown a tantrum of their own. Maybe they hadn't realised they were being so lackadaisical. She wondered if Spira was like every other hospital she'd ever worked at—with a gossip grapevine that spared no one. Could it be they'd realised their own practices were now being discussed by others?

Addy almost groaned out loud. She hadn't thought through all the idiosyncrasies and egos of simply trying to improve practice. With hindsight, it was probably because she didn't know everyone yet. If she'd taken some time to get to know people, she might have realised who to tread carefully with in order to get what she wanted.

But, in the meantime, that would have left patients at risk. And that just wasn't on her game card.

She turned back to the HR director, wondering if this poor woman had had to listen to some consultant ranting and raving about her. 'Thank you,' she said with a nod before walking down the corridor, through the double doors and onto the other ward.

If the other staff knew she was coming they were very easy about it. The ward clerkess immediately gave her a smile. 'Charge Nurse Bates, come and I'll show you where to store your bag, and then I'll show you the office.'

This ward was practically a mirror image of the other, but Addy smiled sweetly and let herself be shown around. She then spent an hour asking the various nurses on duty to give her a rundown of their patients and any immediate issues.

She took some time to talk to the two physio-therapists allocated to the ward, then arranged to meet the ward pharmacist. If she'd still been at home, in an NHS hospital, all of these people would have been the same from ward to ward.

But Spira mainly had people allocated to one ward only. Which then made her wonder about Layla. She'd told her she worked between both wards. Had she managed to upset one of the consultants on the other ward too?

Once she'd finished talking to the staff, she went back into her office. It was clean and tidy, and it appeared that the other charge nurse had moved out their things—or perhaps someone had done that for them.

The desk opposite hers had a computer set up, an odd-looking mug and a half-eaten packet of biscuits. But the rest of the place was pristine.

'Maysa,' she called to the ward clerkess. 'Do I share this office space with someone?'

Maysa smiled at her. 'All of our consultants have their own offices, but some like to work on the ward while they're here.' She raised her eyebrows at the desk. 'The biscuits belong to Theo. He always says he likes to do things right away, in case he forgets.'

Addy wrinkled her nose. 'Why would he forget anything?'

Maysa kept smiling. 'He just has so much on his mind all the time, being on his own with Max and having to learn about being a parent.'

Addy blinked. 'What do you mean…learn about being a parent?'

Maysa's head tilted to the side. 'Oh, he hasn't said anything? Of course you've not really been working with Theo yet. Max isn't his biological child. He's his friend's child, and she died a number of months ago. Theo is Max's godfather, and he took on the role of parent after Max's mother died. They are such an adorable pair.'

Something clicked in her brain from the other night. Max had called Theo by his name. Not Papa or Dad. Theo. She hadn't thought much of it at the time, but it had obviously lingered in her head.

'I live right next to them.' It came out before she had time to think about it.

'You do? That's nice.' Maysa gave her a curious look. 'Do you have any experience with kids? Theo is always looking for advice. He was kind of thrown in at the deep end.'

'He didn't spend much time with Max before?'

Maysa gave a small shrug. 'He showed me a picture of him holding Max when he was younger. I don't think he lived close by his friend, but he definitely visited. Max seems comfortable with him. I'm not really sure what the circumstances were.'

Even though her brain instantly wanted to know everything, she was trying not to ask too many questions. She'd assumed that Max was Theo's son. She'd also assumed there was a mother somewhere in the mix.

Maysa shook her head. 'Anyway, Theo comes in here often. Omar Iqbal comes in too. He's very nice. Lovely family.'

Addy pressed her lips together in a smile. 'Thanks, Maysa.' It was clear if she wanted to know anything, she just had to ask Maysa. She also realised that the whole ward would know she lived near Theo and Max by the end of the shift.

It was odd. That whole short episode in Theo's house had been replaying in her brain for the last few days. At times she wondered if she was misremembering things. But she was sure there had been a few moments when their eyes had caught—when something had buzzed in the air between them.

It was stupid. She had just got here. And the last thing she needed was any kind of flirtation or hint of a relationship. But she couldn't pretend Theo wasn't attractive. She couldn't pretend that French accent didn't wake up parts of her body she'd vowed would remain dead for a while. And no one could ignore Max. He was definitely a cute kid.

What kind of single guy took on their friend's kid on their own?

She contemplated if she'd have the guts to do the same, but, thankfully, she'd never been in that position.

She carried on with her work, completing off-duty for the coming month and looking over some of her staff's previous appraisals. She'd taken a few notes with ideas for staff development, but she wasn't quite sure who to run them past. Maybe the HR director could point her in the right direction now they were on more familiar terms?

The events of this morning started to edge away at her. She'd kept a handle on things, but secretly she was annoyed. While most of the staff she'd worked with in her life were good human beings, she'd come across the occasional misogynistic, chauvinistic person who thought they were better than everyone else. Who talked down to those around them and expected the world to jump at the snap of their fingers.

Thankfully this breed of person was slowly but surely disappearing in hospitals, but it seemed that Spira might still have a few hidden among their ranks.

She would have liked to think that the HR director would have told the potential person to wind their neck in when they'd approached her about Addy. But it seemed not so. This was likely someone who could cause a fuss, and staff around them had spent most of their time placating them. Didn't people realise that this only encouraged their behaviour?

The more she thought about it, the angrier and more indignant she became. She knew she had to temper her annoyance. She was brand new in this role, and it might even be that the person who'd complained about her had wanted her dismissed. The last thing she should do was to behave in any manner that might give them an excuse to be rid of her.

Addy had always conducted herself in a professional manner at work, and she had no intention of changing that.

The door opened and Theo walked in, talking on the phone to someone. 'Can I get that chest X-ray done urgently, please? I need to know for sure if this patient is in a degree of heart failure, or if there's anything else marring the clinical picture.'

His presence in the room made her catch her breath. She tried not to notice how handsome he was, or the way her body seemed to react to the smell of his aftershave.

He looked up in surprise at Addy. 'What are you doing here?' he asked as he finished the call.

She raised her eyebrows. 'You mean you haven't been part of the plot to destroy me?'

He sagged down into the seat across from her with a look of bewilderment on his face. At least that was a good thing.

'I've not been here long enough to plot anything,' he said easily. 'I'm not important enough, and I don't have enough hours in the day. But…' He took a breath and looked amused. 'I might be up to plotting some kind of coup at a later date.'

She leaned forward. 'And why would that be?'

He leaned back and folded his arms. 'Let's just say I'm watching and waiting. Biding my time.'

'Are you planning on becoming leader of the world?'

He shook his head and grinned at her. 'You forget I have a three-year-old. Leader of the world is tame. He'd expect me to be leader of the universe.'

She was struck by the words he'd just said, and what Maysa had just told her. He didn't sound like a new parent. He sounded like an old hand. Maybe he'd just taken to his life change a whole lot better than she had.

'Okay.' She nodded in agreement. 'If that's what Max wants, it's your job to get it.'

He gave a small smile and looked at her again. 'Seriously, what are you doing here?'

She sighed and held up her hands. 'I've been moved. It's apparently to help me settle in.'

She saw something flash across his face. 'Oh,' was all he said.

'That's it? Oh?' Her tone was more annoyed than she meant it to be.

He pulled a face. 'I did wonder how you and Dr Gemmill might get on.'

'So, it was Dr Gemmill who complained about me?'

He held up one hand. 'Hey, hold on. I don't know if *anyone* complained about you.'

'Well, someone has. That's why I've been moved.' She took another breath and tried to be more reasonable, definitely not wanting him to notice the tears that were threatening to prick at her eyes. 'Well, that and the fact I put some papers into the clinical governance committee, suggesting new processes for the cardiac speciality.'

He let out a small laugh. She could tell he was shocked. 'You mentioned that the other day. I take it you ran it past the rest of the staff first?'

She gulped. 'Is that how you normally do things around here?'

This time he raised his eyebrows at her. 'You know that old saying about bringing others along with you on the journey?'

She shook her head. 'Nope. Exactly how old is that saying?'

He laughed while shaking his head. 'If you wanted to change a protocol, a process or write a new standard operating procedure at your last place, how did you do it?'

She frowned. 'It was easy. I revised the protocol or process, asked a colleague to check what they thought, and then I just sent it in to the clinical governance committee.'

'You didn't need to have a whole load of meetings first, to get everyone's opinion?'

She shook her head. 'The clinical governance committee was very inclusive. They would discuss the papers, then send them out to everyone who'd potentially be affected for comment. People would send back some thoughts, or make tracked changes to the document, and it would come back to the group for further discussion and approval.'

She could tell from the look on his face that things didn't happen like that here. Addy put her head in her hands and groaned. 'I take it it's not so straightforward here?'

He let out a sigh and ran his fingers through his dark hair. 'Well, it should be. But some people don't like change.'

She flung up her hands. 'All I'm asking for is safe planning for known patient admissions.'

'I get it, and I agree, but...'

'But?' She could feel herself becoming defensive, but she knew she had to speak up.

'But try and build those relationships first. I'm sure you could be persuasive if you want to be. There's more than one way to do things.'

Addy was definitely annoyed. She was always passionate about work and doing the right things for her patients. 'So, I should pussyfoot around someone who should be better about planning?'

A deep frown creased Theo's brow. 'Pussyfoot?'

She stood up in frustration. 'Tiptoe around them instead of getting straight to the point.'

He nodded. 'I get what you mean, but not everything needs to be a battle.'

She shook her head. 'You tell me you agree with me, but then backtrack with just about everything else you say. Do you want patients to be safe or not?'

The words came out, and she realised how they sounded. Theo shifted his position in the chair and she cringed. She'd likely just annoyed him. 'Of course I do. And I don't follow the same practices as he does. You've brought attention to it now. I bet most of the other consultants had no idea he was being so casual about things. It will go through the clinical governance process and it will likely be approved.'

She was beginning to regret her move. 'I can't sit on things that I think should be improved. I'm always on the side of the patients.'

'As you should be, but I still think you need to try and get to know some of the staff around here.'

She narrowed her gaze, but he dropped his voice. 'If you took some time, you might see that the key person here is Dr Gemmill's secretary. She's a really nice person. If you told her that him casually phoning to say a patient is coming in with no real details is unsafe, she could probably fill in most of the gaps.'

'It doesn't stop his bad practice. What does he learn if I do that?'

Theo stood up and her heart sank. She was being too pedantic. Did she really need to make this point to a brand-new colleague that she was hoping to get on with professionally?

'You're right,' he said. 'What does he learn? But the likelihood is he won't be here much longer. He's been making noises about retiring. Going to his secretary would be the quickest fix.'

'There's other things.' The words were out before she could stop herself.

She could tell he was trying to be careful. 'Other improvements?'

'Yes and no. Staff development. There doesn't

seem to be any kind of rota system for professional development.'

'What do you mean?

'Within cardiology, we have the two wards, the cardiac ICU and the cardiac theatre.'

He frowned. 'But they're all specialisms.'

'And you work in all three. Why don't our other staff have that opportunity?'

She could see the recognition in his eyes. 'You think they should?'

'I think it might be good if that opportunity was there for staff.'

'You'd have to clear it with the theatre charge nurse, and the charge nurses in ICU.'

'Would you be opposed to it?'

He paused. Then, 'No.'

'But? I sense there is a "but".'

'But some consultants might be wary about having staff in Cardiac Theatre who aren't familiar with procedure.'

'I get that. But what happens when they get a new member of staff? Aren't they allowed a period of time to become familiar with the processes?'

'I guess so. I've only been here three months, and all the staff I've met so far are extremely competent.'

'I hear what you're saying. Let me think about it a bit longer, and then I'll meet the other charge nurses and try to come up with a plan. Just think… in a year's time we might have staff who've worked in all three areas and could help anywhere if required.'

She could feel the enthusiasm building inside her—even if Theo wasn't entirely convinced.

He looked at her carefully. 'I've only been here three months and I'm still learning things. Give yourself a chance to get familiar with the place and the people. Then, if you see something you want to change, talk to me. Maybe we could do it together?'

She knew he was trying to be helpful. And while his French accent was soothing, things still felt a little hierarchical. 'You mean a doctor can change things, but a nurse can't?'

He sighed. For the first time she noticed how tired his brown eyes looked. Maybe he'd had a bad night with Max?

He walked to the door, turning before he left. 'No, what I mean is it would be better if we worked together, that's all.'

He disappeared and she sat back down with a thud. Was this what her work life was going to be like now?

She realised how defensive she'd been. She was annoyed about the move and was taking things out on him.

It was unfair, and she knew that. That was part

of being new—she didn't have a friend she could vent to yet. To moan with about the day-to-day things in the workplace that meant very little, but could irk a lot. Theo was the only person she'd even made friendly overtures to. Why was she now trying to push him away?

Her stomach gave an uncomfortable roll. Maybe this was for the best?

The underlying feeling of attraction towards Theo was making her question herself. She didn't want or need someone to flirt with. She really just had to focus on doing her job.

And if doing her job made Theo fall out with her? So be it.

CHAPTER FIVE

IT HAD BEEN an uneasy few weeks. Theo was doing his best to spend his hours at work concentrating on the job, and his hours at home concentrating on Max.

But it seemed like Addison Bates was drifting through both parts of his life like some kind of cartoon ghost. It felt like every time he blinked, she was there.

On the ward, talking to the charge nurses in ICU, with patients and in the office at work. Then, there was the long corridor at home, the elevator, the nearby shops, the gym and the running track at the park.

They were being civil to one another. And things were fine. Except for the undercurrent that was still there between them.

Occasionally he'd catch her eye. Both would look away quickly, but it always seemed like a zap from above. Something he was purposely trying to avoid.

Theo sighed as he packed up things for him

and Max. Today they were going out together. Dubai had a multitude of places to visit for leisure, entertainment and learning. Spira frequently offered discounted tickets to many popular attractions. Theo had already taken Max to two of the adventure theme parks, and a water park. Today he was trying something educational—the Museum of the Future.

They took the Dubai Metro to the unusual oval torus-shaped building set upon a green hill. 'What's that?' asked Max as soon as he spied the glass and metal building.

'That's where we're going today,' said Theo.

He glanced at his ticket. Every ticket allocated a time, but it looked like they would still have to queue. He made sure Max's baseball hat had the flap out at the back to cover his neck as they walked over.

They'd only been waiting a few minutes when they heard a slightly awkward voice behind them.

'Hey, guys, fancy seeing you here.'

'Chocolate lady!' said Max, before Theo even managed to turn around.

Addy was wearing a beige shirt dress, and was already kneeling down to talk to Max by the time he shrugged off his backpack. 'Hey.'

She looked up at him through her dark lashes and he remembered which old-school actress his mother had admired: Elizabeth Taylor. It was

Addy's flawless skin, and definitely the colour of her eyes, that sent a jolt of recognition. Of course Addy had a much more modern hairstyle, but it brought a smile to his face.

'What are you doing here?'

She kept talking to Max. 'It's Addy, but I'll answer to chocolate lady if you want.' She stood up and gave a slightly embarrassed shrug. 'I guess the same as you. Spira gave me discounted tickets, and I don't want to spend any time in the mall in case I spend all my earnings.'

She looked up at the unusual and impressive building. 'Have you been here before?'

He shook his head. 'I think it might all be a bit too old for Max, but we'll give it a go. Something to pass the day and keep us out of the heat.'

She glanced up to the sun as the queue shuffled forward a little. 'I wasn't really expecting to queue, I thought with the timed ticket you would just walk right in.' She looked down at Max and Theo could almost read her mind.

'Complete sunblock,' he said quickly. 'And the rest of the queue is in the shade so we should be fine.'

Thankfully, this wasn't quite as awkward as work. 'Well,' said Addy, 'you've got a three-month head start on me, so after the museum what else can I do on my days off?'

'I'm not sure my recommendations will work for you.'

The queue shifted forward. 'Why's that?' she asked lightly.

She was different out of work—more relaxed. Not hampered by worry about standards, staff and patients. Was it wrong to think that he liked this version of her best?

'Because my recommendations consist of theme parks for kids. We've gone to two so far. Plus a waterpark.'

She half-pulled a face. 'I don't mind theme parks, but I'm not a waterpark fan. I'm too pale and burn too easily. It's just not worth it for me.' She glanced over at Max. 'What did you do with the wee man?'

She said it so casually she obviously didn't give it a second thought. But when he burst out laughing she looked around, as if looking for the source of his amusement.

'The wee man?' he said. 'You sounded so Scottish there.'

Her hand gently tapped his arm. 'I hate to remind you, but I am Scottish, and that is just one of my many turns of phrase.'

'I like it,' he said approvingly. 'Makes you sound like the guy in the ancient Scottish police TV series that my *maman* and *papa* used to watch. They dubbed it with a French translator who still had a Scottish accent.'

'Oh, no.' She shook her head. 'That just sounds so wrong. And, anyhow, the original series was the best. You should listen to it in its pure form. Even some of our English counterparts weren't quite sure what was being said.'

'Oh, I've looked online. I loved the way the main guy said *mhurrr-der...*' He mimicked the Scottish accent, but it was still infused with his own French one and Addy couldn't stop laughing.

'*Mhurrr-der,*' she said helpfully, her Scottish accent identical to the TV show.

'You win,' he said, shrugging in defeat and shooting her a wide smile, then pointed back at Max. 'The "wee man", as you call him, had one of those swimsuits that covers him from neck to toe, and a hat. So, there was no burning. We only stayed for a few hours.'

They'd reached the entrance to the museum now and were hit with a welcome blast of air conditioning. 'Finally,' he breathed as they scanned their tickets and made their way inside the very modern building.

'Mind if I hang around with you both?' Addy asked.

The words had just been forming on his lips to invite her to do the same. 'No problem,' he said quickly and gave Max's hand a squeeze. 'We'd like that, wouldn't we?'

'Will there be ice cream?' asked Max.

Addy laughed. 'Oh, I think I can stretch to buying us all an ice cream.' She smiled as Max held out his other hand to her.

What on earth had she got herself into? Things all seemed so simple in her head. She'd met her colleague and neighbour by accident, and since they were both at the same place, and didn't have any other company, it made sense for them to stick together.

The building was big, consisting of seven floors. Three of those focused on ecosystems, bioengineering, outer space, resource development and health and wellbeing, while other parts were dedicated to young ones. Most of it was over Max's head.

There were other exhibits on health, water, energy and future technologies, but the best floor for Max was the one dedicated for children.

They'd followed other people and started on floor six, working their way down, but it seemed like it hadn't been the best idea.

Theo looked relieved when they reached the kid's floor. 'I did suspect this place might be a bit too old for Max,' he said. 'But I guess I didn't realise quite how much wouldn't be interesting to him.'

He looked disappointed and she got a weird feeling in the pit of her stomach. What must this be like for him? The ward clerkess had told her that he'd taken responsibility for Max unexpectedly, and that he sometimes looked for advice. Plus, he was on his own with the little guy. Being a single parent was tough enough without being thrown in at the deep end.

'Come on, Theo,' she said encouragingly. 'There has been something at every exhibit that he could play or interact with. And it's not like we've spent a long time at those. Once Max has played with what's there for him, we've moved along.'

He groaned and waved his hand to the floor in front of him. 'But I probably should have brought him straight here.'

Addy put one hand on her hip. 'Has Max looked bored to you at any point? Has he complained? Or asked to move along?' She shook her head. 'No, he hasn't. As for this,' she smiled, 'now it's time to let him run loose, and for us to follow his lead.'

She was feeling little twinges that she really didn't want to feel. It was clear how passionate he was about doing a good job parenting Max—

and she wondered how that might impact on any other relationships he could have.

This floor was designed around future heroes letting kids play a part in a game. It might have been a little bit advanced for a three-year-old, but Theo and Addy played alongside him to keep him entertained.

Finally, they were all exhausted. 'How about something to eat?' asked Theo, pointing at the elevator to the restaurants on the seventh floor.

Max was starting to tire, so he carried him in his arms until they picked a restaurant set in the rooftop garden with a nice breeze. He applied more sunscreen to Max, even though they were in a shaded area.

They sat back and perused the menu. 'Spaghetti bolognaise or cheese and tomato pizza?' Theo asked Max.

Max put his finger to his mouth and looked thoughtful. Addy honestly thought she'd never seen a kid look so cute.

Kids have never been on her radar. She didn't mind them. She'd babysat on occasion for friends and she quite liked playing 'auntie'. It meant she got to do all the fun stuff without the hard commitment of rules and parenting. There had been an occasion when one of her friends had been broken from lack of sleep with her new baby and

Addy had offered to take the colicky baby overnight to let her friend get some undisturbed rest.

She'd spent most of the night pacing, listening to the heartbreaking high-pitched cry, and realised exactly why her friend looked exhausted. To be honest, it had put her off for a bit. But she'd never taken the time to really consider having a family. She guessed it had always been in the back of her head that she might like to have one at some point. But with all the drama about her fiancé and the debts, there had just been no time to consider anything.

But now, sitting here with Max, for the first time, she thought about it.

She was thirty-two now. She'd never considered her biological clock ticking. But how long would it be before she could trust someone again? Right now, that seemed like never. What if she didn't meet someone that she could form a relationship with? Would she be brave enough to be a single parent like Theo?

She blinked. Imagining the costs of requiring a sperm donor and IVF. She would likely never be in a position to afford any of those costs—at least not while she still might be fertile enough to produce viable eggs.

She felt a nudge at her elbow and realised the waiter was next to them. 'A glass of pinot grigio, some sparkling water, and the pepperoni and honey pizza, please,' she said quickly, pushing away the thoughts that had filled her head in the blink of an eye. Sometimes she scared herself.

Theo ordered for himself and Max, then relaxed back into his chair. 'Good view,' he said, looking around them.

She nodded in agreement. 'Not quite as good as the apartments though. I sometimes feel as if we sleep amongst the stars.'

He gave her a smile. 'Been brave enough to sleep without blinds?'

She grinned. 'The first night. Do you try to look around to see if anyone can see in?'

He nodded. 'There's nothing quite so creepy as thinking someone might actually watch you sleep, is there?'

She shuddered and laughed. 'And then you realise that no one in the world is interested. What could they possibly have to gain? So you lie there, looking at the black sky and twinkling stars, and it feels a bit like camping as a kid.'

'You camped?' He seemed surprised.

'Didn't everyone?' She wrinkled her nose. 'Or was that just in Scotland?'

He smiled again. 'Not, that was France too. We definitely camped.'

She opened her hands. 'Don't get me wrong. I'm an appliance girl. I like electrical sockets. And home comforts. But I have, on occasion, lain on a blown-up mattress, in a field somewhere, and looked up at the stars.' She raised her eyebrows. 'Until it rained of course.'

He gave her a good-humoured smile. 'You don't like the sound of the rain on your tent?'

Her eyebrows raised mockingly. 'And then you put your hand up to touch the inside of the tent and it's wet? Shortly followed by the deluge?'

He laughed out loud. 'Should have bought a better tent.'

'Should have stayed at home,' she said quickly, raising her wine glass to him.

There was something so nice about this. Max was drawing with some crayons that the waiter had brought them. Theo was slowly sipping a cool beer, and Addy's wine was refreshing and light. They were shaded from the bright sun, and the breeze around them helped keep them cool.

Addy looked around at their surroundings and let out a small laugh. 'If you'd told me six months ago I'd be working in Dubai, looking at this view, and having lunch at the top of a museum, I'd have thought you were writing a work of fiction.' She gave him a soft smile. She didn't need to say the words for him. She knew his life had changed in unimaginable ways too.

His brown eyes went automatically to Max's blond head—he was still colouring. Green apparently was his favourite colour. Theo let out a long sigh. 'Me too,' he agreed, but the look in his gaze was affectionate. 'We all wish we could go back and change things sometimes. But what's done is done. And I'm not sorry that I'm here.'

His gaze met hers. Even though she'd just had a drink, her mouth felt dry. Was he being philosophical, or direct?

There was a zing in the air. And she wasn't imagining it. The breeze wasn't making her skin prickle. His gaze was.

It would be so easy to think he was looking back over his life and just saying he was glad he had Max. But the words seemed a bit different. When he'd said, 'I'm not sorry that I'm here,' it had been as if the 'with you' might have been unspoken, but seemed to be hanging in the air between them.

And it didn't matter how much she told her skin not to tingle. Or how her brain kept telling her any kind of relationship was the last thing she needed—those dark brown eyes of his seemed to pull like an invisible string across the table.

She gave a little cough and picked up her glass again, raising it towards them. 'Me either,' she added quickly, hoping she wouldn't be asked to qualify what that actually meant.

Thankfully the waiter arrived, setting down pizzas for them all. Max happily started eating, then chatting with his mouth partly full about his favourite movie with little yellow creatures in it.

'Slow down,' said Theo, leaning over him and putting a hand on his shoulder. 'Don't talk with your mouth full. You'll have plenty of time to tell Addy the story.' He looked over. 'At least, I think you will. Are you in a rush?'

Something washed over her. It was the oddest thing and seemed to come out of nowhere. Was she in a rush? No. Last time she'd been in a rush it would have been sorting out one of the many disasters she'd been left with back home. But here?

It was a sweeping sensation of loneliness that almost took her breath away. She was here today through pure chance and good luck. If she hadn't met Theo and Max she would have spent the whole day on her own. She'd been here just over three weeks now, and she still hadn't really had a chance to make any friends.

Dubai was a wonderful place, but everywhere she looked people were busy—laughing, chatting, exercising—and it made her feel even more lonely.

But lonely was safe, she reminded herself. If she was lonely, she wasn't being taken advantage of, or manipulated. She had to keep reminding herself of that.

'I'm not in a rush,' she finally answered, looking down and concentrating on her pizza. The last thing she wanted to do was let him know she was embarrassed by the answer. But Max's little hand brushed against hers.

He beamed at her, and she realised he'd finished his pizza, and wanted to tell her the whole movie story. So, she finished her pepperoni and honey pizza and sipped her wine while she listened to his tale. It was clear the yellow creatures were favourites.

'How many movies are there?' she asked Theo.

His brow furrowed. 'I don't know. Six? Seven? Feels like about one hundred.'

'There's another one soon!' Max beamed. 'You should come with us.'

Theo made a strange sort of sound. 'Now, Max, we can't assume that Addy will be free to come to the movies with us. She might be working, or have plans with friends.'

The little slightly sticky hand slid into hers. 'But we're your friends, aren't we, Addy?'

'Of course,' she agreed quickly, acknowledging the little ache in her heart.

She had to try harder. She had to put herself out there in the world. Sealing herself off because of how Stuart had treated her wasn't a long-term solution.

Theo's words made her realise she might not be welcome to join them. Maybe she hadn't even

been welcome today and had just been too un-
aware to pick up on the signals.

He'd been trying to give her an easy get-out
clause. She should take it. And take the hint in
general.

'I've had a great time today, Max. And I've
loved seeing the museum with you. But Theo
is right. When your next favourite movie comes
out, I could be working or have other plans. And
I'd hate for you to miss out. So, you go ahead
with Theo, and maybe you can tell me all about
it some other time?'

Kids weren't subtle. And she could see the
hint of confusion and hurt in his face. 'Okay,' he
said unsteadily, his gaze flicking between her
and Theo.

Theo's face was steady. He waved his hand
to get the check and paid before she even had a
chance to offer.

Five minutes later they were outside the museum. She knew that Theo and Max would head
towards the metro and, although that had been
her plan too, she didn't want it to seem like she
was trying to stay around them.

'I have a little shopping to do,' she said.

Theo gave her a nod.

'I want to add some colour to the apartment.
Put my own mark on it.'

He hadn't asked her for an explanation, so she

wasn't quite sure why it seemed important to justify her shopping arrangements.

She bent down in front of Max. 'I've had a lovely time. Thank you for letting me hang around with you today.'

Before she straightened up, Max reached over and touched her face. The unexpected move instantly made her recoil, but Max still smiled at her. 'Thank you, Addy,' he said.

Theo bent down and swooped Max up into his arms. 'Sorry,' he muttered hurriedly.

But it was her that felt embarrassed. Max had just been doing what three-year-olds do. Why had things suddenly got so awkward?

She stood up, conscious of the heat rushing into her cheeks. 'No problem,' she said, trying to keep her voice light. 'I'll see you guys later.'

And with a wave of her hand, and no idea where she was going, she rushed off.

CHAPTER SIX

THEO GROANED AS his pager buzzed, knowing what it would be without even looking.

He sighed as he picked it up. Yep. Another colleague off sick.

It seemed that half the hospital had picked up some sort of bug. Public and environmental health were currently investigating. No one knew yet if it were some kind of norovirus or gastroenteritis, or where the origins lay. Their Accident and Emergency department was also full of patients from surrounding areas.

'Another one?' asked Maysa as she walked in.

He nodded. Maysa picked up her phone. 'I'll let Addy know. She's trying to keep both wards staffed, and Cardiac Theatre. One of the charge nurses from Cardiac ITU just phoned in too.'

Theo groaned. He'd been keeping his fingers crossed all week that Max wouldn't pick anything up. Some of the children in the daycare had been affected, and these things spread like wildfire around children. He couldn't be at the hospital, and taking care of a sick child, and he wasn't quite sure what he would do.

Well, actually he did know. He would phone in sick too.

The ward phone rang and Maysa answered, looking into the office where Theo was sitting, just as Addy came through the double doors, pager in one hand, notepad and pen in the other.

Theo looked up as Addy came into the room. 'Everything covered for you?'

'Almost,' she said, pulling a face. 'What about you?'

He groaned. 'Another two doctors off sick, but I have cover for the next few days at least.'

There was a slightly awkward pause between them. It had been this way since their day together at the science centre. Theo couldn't quite work out if he or Max had upset or offended Addy in some way, but the friendly, relaxed manner between them had been stilted these last few days, and neither one of them appeared to understand it.

Theo wondered if she didn't want to appear too friendly at work. People did talk. And that was the last thing they both needed. Particularly when any chat would be unwarranted.

But Addy had stuck in his brain. Max had asked after her a few times, even checking if Theo had replaced her chocolate ice cream—which, embarrassingly, he hadn't.

She'd seemed happy during lunch. He'd caught the affection in her eyes for Max, and it had filled him with relief. He'd had friends before who were never relaxed around children, and that made things awkward for everyone. In the past, he'd been on the sidelines, either trying to placate a worried parent, or a nervous and short-tempered friend. Now he was the main event. Max would always be by his side, and he was conscious that he never wanted to put anyone in a position where they might be uncomfortable.

He didn't even know Addy's past. She might have been married. She could have had fertility issues of her own. Or she might consciously have decided she never wanted a family. They weren't close enough to have those kinds of conversations, which left him with a world of questions that circled around and around—especially late at night.

He tried to reexamine everything he'd said, wondering if he'd made her feel unwelcome in any way. If he had it hadn't been intentional. But the truth was he couldn't remember every word he'd said. He just knew that something seemed to be a little off between them right now.

It shouldn't matter. It shouldn't bother him. They were neighbours and work colleagues. That was it.

But it did. It made his stomach squirm in an

uncomfortable way he hadn't experienced in years. Because he couldn't remember being interested in someone like this in a while.

Maysa knocked on the open door. 'I think you're both going to be needed,' she said, with a grave look on her face.

'What?' asked Theo promptly.

'A VIP downstairs in Accident and Emergency. Chest pain, dehydrated, and suffering from diarrhoea and vomiting the last few days.'

Theo frowned. Usually one of their junior doctors covered the floor in Emergency. But it wasn't unheard of for a VIP to ask for a consultant. He'd only met an extremely rich oil man and an international rugby player so far, both of whom had been regarded as VIPs when they'd attended with cardiac symptoms.

'They're certain it's cardiac and not just dehydration?' he asked as he stood.

Maysa pressed her lips together. 'It's not them that's certain. It's the patient.'

Both Theo and Addy looked up.

Maysa shrugged her shoulders. 'It's Dr Gemmill.'

Theo looked directly at Addy. 'Come down with me.'

She put her hand to her chest. 'What? Me? No way. He hates me. I'll only make whatever symptoms he has worse.'

Theo shook his head. 'Who's covering the cardiac theatre?'

She closed her eyes for a second, realising where this was going. 'Me,' she admitted. 'Everyone else has phoned in sick or has sick family members they can't leave.'

Theo's gaze met hers. 'Then if I need to take him straight to Theatre, it's best if you're with me.'

Addy didn't pretend to hide her groan, but she nodded and followed him down the corridor.

Theo knew he was being logical about this. If his colleague was unwell, he didn't want to waste time.

They reached Accident and Emergency in record time. One of the staff gave them a nod of acknowledgement and pointed towards a room at the side.

Theo could hear Dr Gemmill's voice before they even reached the doorway. He wasn't renowned for his good manners.

'Dr Gemmill,' said Theo as he walked into the room, smiling at the nurse who'd clearly drawn the short straw. He watched the monitor's electronic picture of Dr Gemmill's heart for a few seconds. Then he picked up the twelve-lead ECG that had already been performed.

Dr Gemmill took this as his cue to talk. 'You?

There's no one else on duty?' The creases on his brow deepened. 'And what's she doing here?'

'Addy is likely to be assisting me in Cardiac Theatre this evening, since all other staff are sick,' said Theo, keeping his temper in check and his voice steady.

Addy looked over his shoulder. 'Non-stemi,' she murmured, recognising the type of heart attack Dr Gemmill had suffered at a moment's glance.

Theo tried not to smile. He'd known she was good, and he suspected he was about to find out just how good.

'Can you see if the lab results are available?' he asked.

'They're not,' snapped Dr Gemmill.

Theo stepped closer to him. For the nearly four months he'd known this colleague, he'd always been quite lean. But today his skin was papery, waxy and almost looked as if it had collapsed in on itself.

Theo glanced at the IV running on the other side of the bed. 'Can you turn that up?' he asked Addy, as she searched on one of the nearby tablets for the blood results.

Her hand reached out and she upped the rate in a few seconds.

'Do you want to give me some history?' Theo asked Dr Gemmill. He could see on the chart his first name was Alan, but he knew better than to use it. 'You're clearly very dehydrated. How many days have you been unwell?'

'Just treat my MI,' growled Dr Gemmill. 'That's what you're here for.'

'If I don't like your blood results, I won't be taking you to Theatre,' Theo said succinctly. 'I won't take a dehydrated patient who's at risk of further clots or stroke without ensuring you're stable first.'

'We both know what I need,' Dr Gemmill snapped.

Theo nodded. 'After fluids, yes. But not before.'

Addy handed over the tablet. 'Blood results just in.' He wondered if she would try to remain clear of Dr Gemmill, but no. She bent over him. 'Dr Gemmill, let me check your IV site.'

He scowled as she bent over to look at his diminished veins, clearly checking to make sure the fluids were still running in correctly. The veins in patients with dehydration could often collapse.

'Might need another site,' she said softly.

Theo sighed. 'Okay, your cardiac enzymes are consistent with what the ECG shows us. But your urea and electrolytes mean we have to delay Theatre. I'll run them again in half an hour, after we get another IV into you.'

'You'll overload me, you fool!' Dr Gemmill exclaimed.

Theo merely turned the tablet around to show Dr Gemmill his own results. 'I won't overload you,' he said quietly. 'But you clearly have a limited volume circulating right now. If we want your angioplasty and stent insertion to be a success, we have to delay.'

There was silence in the room. Addy moved around and inserted another IV while the doctors looked at each other. She'd run the other IV through, and connected it, before they finally spoke again.

'Would you take a patient with these blood results for stent and angio?'

They both knew the answer was no. And they both knew the older man wouldn't admit it.

'I suspect,' said Theo, 'that you might be unique. You might actually be a patient whose heart attack has been caused by dehydration, rather than atherosclerosis.' He raised his eyebrows slightly at his colleague. 'Although your age goes against you, you have no other real risk factors I can see in your chart—we both know that means little. Any family history?'

'No.'

'Your cholesterol levels have always been good. Ever a smoker?'

'No.'

Theo sighed inwardly. 'Anything else I should know before considering you for Theatre this afternoon? Allergies?'

'None.'

Addy had finished what she was doing and was talking in a low voice to the nurse.

'What are you whispering about over there?' snapped Dr Gemmill.

Theo felt himself bristle. He knew that, right now, Dr Gemmill was likely terrified. He was about to put his life into Theo's hands, and Theo had no doubt that the mere thought was crippling him with anxiety.

The man was arrogant, over-confident and downright rude as a human being. But he was also a patient. Theo's patient. But no matter who he was in this hospital, Theo wouldn't allow him to talk to staff like that.

It turned out Addy could more than handle him. 'You,' she said succinctly. 'We're talking about you, Dr Gemmill. I'm talking with Faizah here about getting a portable chest X-ray arranged, and what time to get your next set of bloods taken. All being well, I'm also giving her some pre-op instructions for you, since I'll have to go and prepare the cath lab.'

She gave Dr Gemmill the sincerest smile.

'Apologies, I would normally stay with a patient to talk them through everything and make sure they were fully prepared for Theatre, but unfortunately, as you know, there's a shortage of staff, and I'm very *particular* about things.' She laid some emphasis on the word 'particular', and then continued. 'I like to ensure everything in my theatre is laid out exactly as I like. I want to ensure everything is perfect.'

Theo could see all the words that Alan Gemmill actually wanted to say bubble beneath his skin. There was nothing wrong with anything Addy had said, or how she delivered it. But Alan Gemmill was no fool.

Addison Bates had just let him know in the nicest possible way that she was no slouch, and he was lucky to be in her hands.

She shot Theo a beaming smile. 'Dr Dubois, I take it I can leave all the consent procedures with yourself while I go and prepare Theatre?' She glanced from Dr Gemmill to Theo. 'Providing of course the future blood results are sufficient.'

He gave her a nod and didn't let himself smile as she left the room in a few strides. Theo glanced at the clock. He turned to Faizah. 'Optimal reperfusion time is ninety minutes for best effect.' He gave her a time. 'Can the bloods be taken then? I'll phone the lab and let them know I need the results fifteen minutes later.'

Faizah nodded.

'Great, then these are the rest of the instructions for Dr Gemmill.' He wrote up some medications and timed observations. Finally, he finished the consent procedures with Alan Gemmill, and asked the most important question.

'Can I call someone for you? A family member or a friend?'

His colleague still had a disgruntled expression on his face. Theo actually wondered if he had anyone. 'I called my wife and left her a message. She hasn't replied yet.'

Theo stopped the million questions that immediately sprang into his head. 'Do you have any idea where she currently is?'

'At her club.' His words were staccato.

'And where's that?'

He murmured an address and Faizah raised her head. 'Oh, I know that place. I know someone who works there. Let me call and see if I can get a hold of her.'

If Theo had blinked he would have missed the tiny movement in Alan Gemmill's shoulders, which might have indicated a little sigh of relief.

Maybe the guy did have some feelings after all. 'Do you have any questions for me, Dr Gemmill?' Theo asked.

The older man shook his head.

'Then I'll go and get scrubbed for Theatre. I'm hoping your blood results will be a bit better and we can get started as soon as possible. If there's a problem, I'll come back and let you know. Otherwise, I'll see you in the cath lab.'

Addy was thanking her lucky stars she'd made a few visits to the cardiac theatre, to meet the charge nurse and get shown around. She'd sown the seeds of her idea of rotating staff, and it had gone better than she'd initially hoped. Luca, the charge nurse down here, had wanted to chat further, and explore how best they could manage things.

However, Luca was currently on a two-week holiday to the US. She suspected if he knew about the sickness levels at Spira right now, he would jump back on a plane, but that didn't help her or Theo today.

She talked to the anaesthetist on call, and to the theatre technician on duty. The theatre was prepared in record time. It wasn't difficult—this was a permanent cardiac theatre, so the main pieces of equipment remained in place.

She looked out the theatre packs, angio lines and stents, before briefing the imaging technician and finally going to change into scrubs.

By the time she was at the theatre sink, Theo was next to her. 'Bloods okay?' she asked.

He nodded. 'Not normal as yet, but improved. Enough that I'm confident to do the procedure.'

'The anaesthetist, Hal, is on standby if you need them.'

Theo gave a nod. 'He said he would have a chat with Dr Gemmill in pre-op to let him know he was available if sedation was required.'

'Does everyone jump to Dr Gemmill's word?'

Theo gave her a sideways glance as he scrubbed. 'No. To be honest, I think Hal would take great pleasure in anaesthetising the guy. Probably wanted to do it for years just to keep him quiet. But that's hardly a thing you can say out loud.'

Addy grinned at his frankness. 'Well, I know the charge nurse down here thinks very highly of Hal. Says if he's ever sick and needs an op, he's calling Hal on his way in.'

'Now, that's praise indeed from a colleague,' said Theo as he dried off his hands. Then they finished gowning and gloving.

Addy stood at his side as Dr Gemmill was wheeled into Theatre and positioned on the table. Theo hadn't been joking when he'd said everything was state-of-the-art here. They had a bi-plane system, which captured 3D images faster because they used detectors on two axes instead of one. It looked like two giant arms shaped like Cs, which could be moved and manipulated around the table where the patient lay.

Dr Gemmill was still scowling, but Addy kept smiling and talking in a reassuring manner as the technician ensured electrodes were placed where they should be and the BP cuff was in place. They were ready to start.

Theo started to talk. His accent was rich and thick. She'd never been in the cath lab with him before, so didn't know if this was his normal manner, or if he might actually be a little nervous.

Treating patients that you knew was always different and sometimes difficult. Addy had been part of the resuscitation of a previous colleague and it had stuck with her—no matter that she knew everything had been done perfectly.

Addy draped the groin area, where Theo would start the procedure. She cleaned it with the orange-coloured antiseptic that was used all over the world, then he injected local anaesthetic to numb the area.

Dr Gemmill was quieter than she'd expected, and she suspected the anaesthetist might have given him something to relax him. It was probably better for everyone.

But whether Dr Gemmill was listening or not, Theo talked him through what he was doing. He made the small incision, inserted the sheath then passed the catheter, watching its ascent as he guided it along the coronary artery.

A thin flexible wire was then inserted down the inside of the catheter once they found the narrowed area in the artery. Theo had been right.

There was little evidence of plaque inside the arteries—which was usually common in patients with cardiac conditions. However, when they reached the left coronary artery, there was clear sign of blockage—a thick clot.

Theo inserted some medicine specially designed to dissolve the clot in a harmless way. Then he inflated the balloon to relieve the blockage and allow the blood to flow through the heart. The tiny stent was already in position. As Theo deflated the balloon, the stent stayed in place as it was designed to.

Dr Gemmill's heart rate remained steady throughout, with only the occasional ectopic beat. Theo finished by inserting some contrast dye to monitor the blood flow through the heart and ensure there were no other blockages.

The whole procedure took just under thirty minutes. The balloon, wire, catheter and sheath were all removed, and Theo applied pressure to the wound, talking comfortably to Dr Gemmill until he was happy the wound was sealed.

They had a short talk about pain relief, future plans and the need for possible antithrombotic medicine in the future. Dr Gemmill was scornful—so he was obviously feeling a bit better—and was confident that dehydration had caused his blockage and he wouldn't require anything else. However, he did accept that Theo would ask him to be reviewed by one of their specialist colleagues to discuss this further before he was discharged from hospital.

When Dr Gemmill was wheeled out through the door, Theo and Addy let out big sighs of relief as they tugged off their theatre caps.

Addy bent down and shook her hair out, tossing it back over her head when she was finished. Her dark, normally smooth hair had some kinks and curls.

'Phew,' she said. 'I've too much hair for these theatre caps. They kill me.'

He laughed at her. 'It does seem to have doubled in size.'

She glanced about, looking for a mirror, but there was none. 'Is it that bad?' She stalked around, patting her inflated hair. 'Humidity. It plays havoc with me. My hair is just too thick. I'll need to find a good hairdresser to help me thin it out.'

Theo had folded his arms and was leaning against a wall. 'Thinning out your hair. That's actually a thing?'

'Of course,' she said, pulling her scrub top free of her trousers and letting it hang. The theatre changing rooms were surprisingly warm.

Theo stuck up his hand to feel the air. 'Think the air conditioning's broken in here?'

She laughed. 'Either that or they spent so much

money on all the equipment they can't afford to turn it on. Maybe they're just trying to stop us all hanging around by making it a sweat-fest in here.'

This was the first time they'd been alone since their day at the science centre. It felt nice again. It felt right. And as soon as that tiny thought entered her head, she could feel the wave of panic circling her again.

'I really need to shower,' she said, heading to her locker to grab her things.

Theo gave a nod at her sudden move. He was watching her carefully, she could tell. 'I'll need to finish up my notes. Are you working on the ward tomorrow?'

She nodded and then her feet stopped. She turned around. 'Is that going to be a problem?'

Theo looked puzzled. 'No. Why? I was only asking for continuity of care.'

But Addy froze. 'You know he doesn't like me. He moved me off his ward.'

Theo moved next to her. 'But I'm his consultant.' He patted his hand against his chest. 'So, he'll have to stay on *my* ward, not his.'

She shook her head. 'He won't want me anywhere near him. And I bet he's a complainer.'

Theo looked at her quizzically. 'You are more than fit for him. That's how you say it, isn't it?'

A smile hinted at her lips. 'Maybe,' she agreed reluctantly. Then she gave a big sigh. 'But he's a cardiac patient who's just undergone a procedure. The last thing I want to do is add any stress. It's probably best I'm nowhere near him.'

'Then try not to be.'

'You know what the staffing is like.'

'I do,' Theo agreed. 'And so does he. I expect you to treat him like every other patient.'

She instantly felt her hackles rise and opened her mouth to answer, but Theo's soft hand rested on her shoulder. 'Like the excellent nurse that you are. You're experienced, have lots of knowledge, and likely know as much as any of us. Don't be intimidated by him. Think of him as one of those patients who are nasty, rude and tetchy because, deep down, they're scared. He's just had a life-threatening event. Right up until his chest pain today, Dr Gemmill probably thought he was going to live for ever.'

She was conscious of the warm feeling of his palm through her thin scrub top. They were inches apart, and the only two in the changing room. The heat wasn't just coming from the air around them. It was coming from inside.

She tilted her head upwards. He was close enough for her to see the tiny scratchy stubble around the edge of his jawline. His brown eyes were a little bloodshot—probably from the pressure of today. But, this close, she could also see just how long his dark eyelashes were. Women would go to war over eyelashes like those.

She could smell him. That cologne that he wore. She'd noticed it a few times. Hints of it were still there—amber, woody, but still fresh. She tried not to suck in her breath. That would just be too weird.

His fingers moved a little, one coming into contact with her skin. There it was—the reaction that she'd known would happen. All of the cells in her body coming alive in instantaneous response. Instead of sucking a breath in, she let a breath out, in an odd kind of sighing way.

In that instant, she saw his pupils dilate, and he leaned towards her.

Neither of them had spoken. They didn't need any dialogue. Their bodies were doing all the talking.

The door swung open behind them and both of them jumped.

The theatre orderly's gaze narrowed for a second, as if he realised what he'd almost seen. Then he said, 'There's a woman outside to see you. Somebody Gemmill. She won't go to the waiting room. Believe me, I've tried.'

A smile broke across Addy's face and she stepped back. It was odd. Her body was on fire, but she now felt strangely relieved.

What would have happened if they'd kissed? It

could be a disaster. They barely knew each other. Addy was here to get her life in order, and she certainly hadn't achieved that yet.

But as Theo stepped back his hand brushed against her bare arm. Only in the slightest way, his fingers making a lightning soft trail down her forearm to her wrist.

The zap was like being hit by a magic wand. The pads of her fingers tingled—as if they were crying out to grab his hand as it drifted away from her skin.

It was the smallest move, and looked almost unintentional, but as Theo walked to the door, she saw his sideways glance at her. 'I'll speak to Mrs Gemmill,' he said, his voice huskier than usual. 'See you back outside.'

And then he was gone. Leaving her more in need of a shower than she had been before.

CHAPTER SEVEN

IT TURNED OUT that Mrs Gemmill was probably the most interesting patient's relative that he'd met in all his years as a doctor.

She was big. She was flamboyant. She was loud. And she was the biggest sweetheart he'd ever met.

Mrs Gemmill wore hats, and they usually matched her lipstick and her shoes. She went to a variety of 'clubs'—most of which Theo was sure he'd never see the inside of.

Addy stood next to him with her arms folded, watching the spectacle at the end of the corridor as Mrs Gemmill said hello to every person, in every room, before reaching her husband.

'She's got to be old money.'

Theo looked at her. 'What do you mean?'

'I mean, I think Alan Gemmill married up. She's a lady. I bet she actually has a title. Have you heard the number of charities she's involved with? She goes to Ascot every year. Wimbledon. She's gone to the Grand Prix in Monaco. And she never boasts. She talks about these things as if they were every-day normal.'

Theo leaned over and whispered in her ear. 'Do you think he ever gets a word in?'

That made Addy grin, her smile spreading across her face. Her violet eyes turned to him. 'You know, I doubt it, and funnily enough, that makes me happy.'

Alan Gemmill had stayed a day longer than usual because it seemed the dehydration was taking a few days to recover. He was a little unsteady on his feet, and his blood pressure was generally low. All in keeping with an older patient who'd had a bug for a few days and become severely dehydrated—and that was all without taking into consideration his MI, angioplasty and stent insertion.

Theo was quite sure the man would have dragged himself out of the ward any way he could, if possible. But it seemed that Mrs Gemmill had some kind of background knowledge herself in medicine, and was happy to go along with Theo's recommendation that Dr Gemmill stay until all his levels were entirely normal and he was fully fit again.

And it seemed that her husband was not getting a chance to overrule her.

'I'm going to bask in these few days,' said Addy as she took a cookie from a huge basket on the desk—also supplied by Mrs Gemmill. 'He snapped at me as I changed his IV, and she put him back in his place in a heartbeat. She was literally mortified by him, and I don't imagine she has any idea how he normally is at work.'

'Did you get a chance to meet Dr Gemmill's secretary when she came down?'

Addy nodded again. 'It seems that she and Mrs Gemmill are in cahoots.'

'Cahoots? What's that?'

She gave a quiet laugh. 'It means they're in an alliance together, a partnership, and it generally means up to no good.'

Theo took a couple of seconds to get his mind around that one, then nodded in approval. 'Maybe that's the only way they manage him.'

Addy turned to face him. They had managed to stay at arm's length for the last two days. Memories of the changing room had flooded his mind at all possible instances, along with the eternal what-if question.

The main focus of the question was central to him and Max. He'd never been a single parent before, he'd never tried to date anyone while he was a single parent. So many things were new to him. Should he have rules? Should he have actually tried to date someone before allowing them to meet Max?

Maybe Max should never meet someone he

dated—unless… He couldn't even think about the unless. It was a million miles away.

Addy knew about Max. She'd met him. She seemed good with him. But he was conscious he didn't know so much about her. He didn't want to take a chance on something that could be fleeting and then damage any future working relationship.

But, as the floral scent of her perfume drifted under his nose, he wondered if fleeting and casual might be the way to go. It had never really been his style. But maybe he could keep any relationship fully at arm's length, and keep Max cocooned from that part of his life. Would that work better? Would that keep Max from making friendships with women that might actually do him more harm than good?

He just wasn't ready for this. For the myriad of what-ifs that had been circling his brain. And this wasn't the kind of thing he could pick up the phone to Colette about. Any Max-related question was fine. But how to have a love life as a single parent? Colette would put him firmly back in his place if he tried to ask for advice on that issue. The thought brought a smile to his face.

'Any chance he might retire now?' asked Addy, her voice hopeful.

Max shrugged. 'I'm his doctor right now, but I don't think he'll want to have the conversation with me about reducing his workload. He's fixating on the fact his MI was likely caused by dehy-dration. I think if he could get away with it, he'd write up his own case for some journal.'

'Why don't you?'

Theo spoke quietly and couldn't keep the smile out of his voice. 'It's unusual but not *so* unusual that I want to tell the world about it. Last time I saw a case like this the guy was in his late twen-ties, fit as a fiddle, and worked in a printing fac-tory where the temperatures were through the roof—and it was in the middle of summer. Now, that case was interesting, and the consultant I worked with at the time wrote it up. This one? Not so much.'

'You don't think Dr Gemmill needs the fame?' Amusement was in those eyes.

'I think that's the last thing he needs.'

She gave a sigh and continued to nibble her cookie. 'His wife's nice. I wonder how he man-aged to catch her.'

'Catch her? Somehow I think if I said that you might give me trouble.'

'Maybe.' She shrugged good-naturedly. 'I just find it fascinating that a person who's a tyrant and a grump at work managed to find such a charm-ing wife.'

'She is charming, isn't she?'

Addy tapped him on the arm. 'But you know what that means now, don't you?'

He was focusing on the tiny spot on his arm that her fingertip had just touched. It was ridiculous how his eyes went there. Or how, when she'd been right in front of him two days ago, close enough to kiss, he could see both shades of blue and violet in her eyes, merging to make that heart-stopping colour. How her skin had been so perfect, even though she'd just taken off her surgical mask. And her hair...oh, her hair brought a wide smile to his face.

'Hey,' she said, nudging him with her elbow. 'Pay attention.'

'Sorry.' He gave himself a shake, trying to pretend his mind hadn't gone to other places.

'You know what this means, right?'

He was bewildered, and still wondering if, even though they were on the ward, they might be standing a little too closely.

'I haven't got a clue.' He sighed, hoping this didn't mean she would move.

She threw up her hands. 'His patients. They're yours right now. Including...' She waited, as if he would throw out the name. But she gave up in exasperation. 'Isabel Aurelis.'

The young girl who had arrested on their first meeting.

'But that was almost a month ago. She was discharged after a few days.'

Addy tapped the side of her nose. 'But her investigations haven't been completed. She still has episodes and symptoms.'

He frowned and looked at her. 'And how would you know that?'

'Layla,' she said promptly. 'She's doing some learning right now, and she's based her patient case on Isabel and her potential condition of Wolff-Parkinson-White Syndrome.'

'I can get away with looking after the patients that Dr Gemmill currently has admitted—or who are scheduled for procedures that shouldn't wait. I don't think I'll get away with calling in one of his private patients.'

'I have contacts.' Addy beamed.

Her hair was back under control, smooth and gleaming under the hospital lights, caught in a burgundy scrunchie that matched her uniform. Theo wasn't sure what way he liked it best.

He groaned. 'Dr Gemmill's secretary.'

'Finally,' she said, throwing up her hands again. 'She'll bring Isabel in if you ask.' Her tone changed, as she clearly tried to make herself sound innocent, as if she hadn't planned this to get Isabel's care reviewed.

He took a breath. 'You are going to get me in all sorts of trouble.'

She winked. 'Hope so.'

It was so easy and natural between them. And

he liked it. He liked being around her. Even when he tried to find reasons not to.

The thought of Addison Bates getting him into trouble did all sorts of things to him that it shouldn't.

He picked up a cookie. 'I will see her *if*, and I mean if, she still has symptoms that need investigating, or *if* she still needs test results explained to her.' He waved the cookie as he walked down the corridor.

'I understand,' Addison said brightly, with a big smile on her face.

And he knew she was indeed going to get him into trouble.

Seven hours later she was sitting on her sofa with the weirdest feeling sizzling in her belly. It was like an itch that she wanted to scratch but didn't exactly know where it was. There were a million things she could watch on TV or streaming services, but it wasn't what she wanted to do.

She started to pace, looking out at the dark sky, the outline of the skyscrapers and the twinkling stars above. Her phone pinged and she sighed as she picked it up. But the sigh was quickly extinguished when she realised who the sender was.

Are you free to come over? I have a debt to repay.

She looked down at her 'lounging' outfit. Soft beige joggers and a matching giant off-the-shoulder sweatshirt. She should change. She should find something more alluring to put on. But as she hurried through to the bedroom and caught a glance of herself in the mirror, she stopped. Some of today's make-up was left in place and her hair was in a half-up, half-down style, because of how she'd been lying on the sofa a while ago. If she changed, how long would that take? And should she really dress up to go practically next door?

She looked down again. Her clothes were fine. Not what she would wear to go shopping, but they were clean, no stains—certainly good enough to go two doors down. She gave herself one panicked spray of light perfume, then grabbed her key and her phone.

He opened the door with a big smile on his face. She was glad she hadn't changed—he was wearing an old shirt, some shorts and a pair of worn-in designer flip flops that he'd probably got in his youth.

'Wine or beer?' he asked.

She looked around. 'Where's Max?'

'Sleeping.' He looked relieved as he said the words. 'It's just us.'

That sent a little tingle to her stomach. 'Wine,' she said. 'White if you have it.'

Two minutes later they were perched on his sofa, looking out at the dark night.

'I was doing this next door,' she said as she sank into the cushions. 'Don't you like to do this?'

He laughed. 'Sometimes it's all I can do.'

'What do you mean?' She turned slightly to face him, letting one of her arms rest on the back of the sofa, her knee pulling up too.

He gave a sigh, but kept smiling. 'By the time I get back from work, collect Max, feed him, bath him, play with him, I just don't have the energy for chat shows or action movies.' He waved his arm at the dark sky through the glass. 'This is as good as it gets.'

'You've turned your sofa to face it,' she said, looking around. 'I like it.'

'Don't get fooled.' He laughed. 'The rest of the time it's definitely facing the TV. Max is a special expert on certain kids' shows.'

She let her head fall back. She felt surprisingly comfortable in here. 'I'll bet he is. What's his favourite?'

'Some guy walking around an empty nursery, playing with the toys and singing.'

She shot him a sideways glance. 'That sounds a little bit creepy.'

Theo laughed too. 'It does, doesn't it? Honestly, it's fine, and he sings along and does all the actions. Nothing dubious. I promise.'

She took a breath and then asked, 'So, how is Max?'

'What do you mean?'

'I mean, he had a big change some months ago. He's with you, you've moved. How's he doing?'

Theo closed his eyes for a few seconds and she wondered if she'd got too personal. But she couldn't deny the attraction between them, and they were becoming friends. It felt right to ask.

His dark brown eyes met hers. He bit his lip before replying. 'He's doing fine. At least I think he is. He has the occasional nightmare, and that freaks me out, because I don't know everything he was exposed to, and all the research now tells us that the first two years of a kid's life are for-mative.'

Addy nodded. She'd heard that too—particu-larly when she'd had to work with traumatised adult patients. She reached out her hand. 'But that doesn't mean you can't shape what comes next.'

He let out a breath and she could sense his body relax a bit more. His hand closed over hers. She shifted a little so she could still drink her wine with her other hand, and it brought their shoul-ders side by side.

'I worry I don't spend enough time with him. I worry that I don't have an extended family here. It feels disloyal to France to bring Fleur's child here and bring him up in Dubai instead of back home.'

'Isn't seeing the world a good way to shape a kid's life experience? You already told me he's bilingual. His English is great.'

Theo shook his head a little but smiled. 'Oh, he keeps his French for when he's having a temper tantrum.' He raised one eyebrow. 'He might know a few phrases that he shouldn't.'

'Does he have many temper tantrums?'

'Not really. I mean, I don't think he has more than any normal three-year-old.'

'Then surely that means you're doing a good job?'

He took a sip of his wine.

She could tell he was still stressed, still worrying. 'And isn't it the job of every parent to always secretly worry?'

She leaned a little bit forward, so she could get a good look at those eyes. Should she actually be worried about Theo?

'I guess so,' he said, but the tone of his words sounded defeated.

'So, how are *you* doing?'

The edges of his lips turned upwards. 'Aren't you supposed to say that like Joey from *Friends*?'

She laughed and made an attempt to mimic the character, then shook her head. 'No, I just can't do it. The Scottish accent is too strong.'

He nodded in agreement, then tilted his head

as he looked at her. 'No one has really asked me that since I took on Max.'

'Then you're hanging around with the wrong folks.' Addy had never been one to beat around the bush.

He gave a sad kind of smile. 'That's not strictly true. My *maman* asks, but she has enough to worry about.'

'What's wrong with your mum?'

He shook his head. 'Not my mum, my dad. He has multiple sclerosis and my mum is his full-time carer. It's partly why I moved to Dubai. When they knew I was going to take care of Max, my parents asked if I wanted to move back home with them. But I knew that was unfair. My mother would have wanted to help out, and she really isn't able. She has enough to deal with, and I didn't want to put any more strain on her, or on them.'

'How's your dad doing?'

'Okay,' said Theo carefully. 'His deterioration has slowed. He can still manage things with as-sistance. I'm hoping that he'll stay like that for a while.'

She could see from his face that she didn't need to ask the next question. Should his father get worse, Theo would want to be there, he would want to go home to France. She didn't blame him at all.

'So, you didn't answer,' she persisted. 'How are you doing?'

He met her gaze, and she could feel the invisible barrier between them. There were a million things he didn't know about her. She wasn't sure she would ever be ready to share—not when her past made her look like a fool. It made her feel so vulnerable, and she didn't want to share that with anyone.

'I hope I'm doing okay,' he said, this time with a bit more confidence. 'Mind you, having to do surgery on a colleague was a bit nerve wracking.'

'You don't say?' she mocked.

'But I'm glad it was you that was there.'

She gestured with her wine glass towards her chest. 'You mean, so I could deflect his bad mood, and keep you safe.'

He smiled but shook his head. 'No, because I know that you know what you're doing. I was confident in the person standing next to me, so it meant I didn't need to worry.'

'Thank you,' she said simply, then leaned forward and whispered in his ear. 'But let's not have a repeat, okay?'

She was so close to his ear that when he turned his face towards her his nose brushed against her cheek. They both froze for a second.

She blinked, conscious that he'd silently set his wine glass down. He reached over and took hers from her hand. Their faces were only inches apart, and she could feel his warm breath next to her cheek.

'Hey, did you get me here under false pretences?' she whispered.

His voice was low. 'What do you mean?'

'You said you had a debt to repay?'

One of his hands moved to her cheek, his fingertips running down the side of her face. He gave her a lazy kind of smile. 'There's a problem with that now.'

'Really?' Her breath was catching in her throat at his touch. 'And what might that be?'

'Well…' it was almost a drawl '…if I repay my debt, we'll both have to move. I kind of don't want to do that right now.' His warm hand moved to her waist, slipping under her loose top and resting on her bare skin.

She smiled and closed her eyes for a second, enjoying the buzz. 'I kind of don't want you to move either, but I still want to know what this debt is.'

His head bent a little, his lips connecting with the soft skin at her neck. She tipped her head back as his mouth explored the area at the bottom of her throat, then moved up to her ear.

His lips touched her ear. 'Chocolate,' he whispered with a laugh. 'We owe you chocolate, and Max reminded me to pay our debt.'

'You bought me ice cream?' Her eyes connected with his. They widened as she challenged him, shifting her hips to move astride him, as his fingers danced up her bare back.

'Yep,' was all he could muster from her change of position. 'Sure you want to do that?'

She arched her back a little towards him. 'Oh, I'm sure. Now,' her fingers drew down one side of his face, 'I hope you got me all the trimmings.'

His dark eyes flashed in confusion, but he couldn't remove the smile from his face.

'What trimmings?'

'You know...' Her fingers moved down the front of his T-shirt, sliding underneath as he caught his breath. 'All the things that Max likes. The chocolate sauce, the sprinkles, the marshmallows.'

Her eyes were sparkling as she said the words, taking delight in teasing him as they spoke. All her previous precautions were dancing out through the window. It was funny how his touch could do that to her.

Scotland was a distant memory. She was miles away from thoughts of debt and betrayal. All she wanted to think about was the here and now. They were both grown-ups. This could be whatever they wanted it to be. She was capable of having some fun with her friend. Everything else could just wait.

'So, you like all the trimmings?' he said again, at the base of her throat.

Her hands moved, tugging his T-shirt over his head, then mimicking the act with her own soft top. She glanced over her shoulder into the dark night. 'Think anyone can see us?' she asked.

'Couldn't really care,' was his muffled reply as he pulled down one strap of her bra, then released the back clasp with the other hand.

She could stop this. She could stop this now if she wanted to.

But she absolutely didn't. Because the only thing on her mind right now was Theo Dubois, and just how good this could be. The anticipation was currently killing her.

She asked one final question as she glanced at the door in the corner. 'Any chance Max might wake up?'

Theo shook his head. 'Even if he has a nightmare, he stays in bed. I go to him. He never comes to me.' His eyes met hers. 'We're safe.'

'Good,' she replied with a grin as she pulled him down sideways, then on top of her. His lips touching hers was like heaven.

She could tell that her breathing was shallow. They had both been waiting for this moment. It meant their first kiss was breathless, in a mad teenage kind of way, which made her instantly smile and think of a million movies. Breathless in a way that made her legs liquid, even though she was lying down.

His teeth were on her lips, his tongue was in

her mouth, and a million blood cells were currently racing around her body.

His chest was against hers and she could swear she could feel both their racing hearts through their skin. The groan that came from the back of his throat almost undid her.

He stopped for a second, as if he were trying to catch his breath. 'Addy.' His voice was a low growl. 'Are you sure about this? We've only known each other a few weeks.'

'Five,' she responded without hesitating, because it was front and foremost in her mind. She didn't care that she'd told herself she wasn't looking for a relationship. She didn't care that they hadn't had the chance to talk about all their past issues. All she cared about was the right here and now. The feel of his warm body against hers. The touch of his hand on the skin at her back.

'What if people ask about us? Notice a change between us?'

She was smiling and in real danger of clashing teeth with him as their kiss deepened. 'Let them wonder,' she breathed, moving her kisses around to his ear. 'Let's keep this here. Between us. We can tell them when we're ready.'

She was sliding her hands to his front, across his chest, then winding her hands around his neck so she could pull him even closer.

'I can live with that,' he said, then lowered his head to make her forget about anything else.

CHAPTER EIGHT

THE REDIRECTED LETTER came like a bolt out of the blue. Her solicitor knew where she'd relocated to, but this letter was from the police, saying a new inspector was in charge of her case, and criminal charges might be brought. She should attend for interview immediately.

It had been sent more than a month ago, and it had finally made its way to her in Dubai. Addy thought she was going to be sick.

She'd spent the last week floating around in a pink bubble, spending as much time as she could with Theo and Max. No one knew that they were dating or in any kind of relationship. Even Addy wasn't quite sure how to define it.

What she did know was the feel of his skin against hers, the touch of his fingers and lips, had cast some kind of spell over her. All she wanted was more. She hadn't stayed overnight at his place yet. But walking the few steps between their apartments in the early hours of the morning was rapidly becoming the norm.

She couldn't remember being this excited or happy at the start of any of her previous relationships. Being around Theo was hypnotic. But her giant pink bubble had just been burst with a letter-shaped pin.

She spent more than an hour trying to get hold of her solicitor. Finally, Laura let out a huge sigh when she heard the news. 'Leave it with me. Let me deal with this.'

'But what does it mean? It was me that spoke to the police about Stuart. It was me that wanted to bring charges against him.'

She heard Laura draw in a deep breath. 'He's reappeared. He's causing trouble. He likely outstayed his welcome wherever he went and thought that things would have blown over back home. He's denying he took out the new mortgage or some of the debts. He's telling the police it was all you, and it doesn't help that his return coincided with the original inspector retiring.'

'But what does that mean for me?'

'Nothing. It means nothing. We know some of the debt was taken online. They have no signatures to prove it was you or an electronic footprint. You gave two previous interviews, which more than covered anything they need to know. Leave me to deal with this. Send me a photo of the original letter.'

Addy could feel the wave of panic coming

over her. The timing could not be worse. She'd just started to settle into life in Dubai, she'd met someone, she'd just taken some tentative steps towards a new relationship—and now this.

'He's a parasite.' Laura's voice cut into her thoughts. 'He doesn't want to be held accountable for his actions. I'm pretty sure he'll just be setting up his next target, and then he'll disappear again.'

'He doesn't know where I am, does he?' Sudden fear had struck into her heart. Stuart had never been physically abusive towards her, but she didn't know what he might do if he was pushed.

There was a brief pause. 'Not as far as I know. Addy, let me deal with this. I promise I'll be back in touch, okay?'

Addy hung up the phone, her heart racing. She dug into the fridge and pulled out a big bowl of fruit salad, sitting at her table and eating her way through it. A sugar rush always helped when she felt like this. And now wasn't the time for the chocolate ice cream Theo had given her the other night.

She leaned her head in her hands. Just when things had started to look good.

With Dr Gemmill still recovering and not at work, some of the tension in the workplace had disappeared. Word on the street was that his wife was in the process of persuading him to take retirement.

Addy was due to hear back from the clinical governance committee next week around her submission, and she was hopeful it might have some feedback she could work with.

As for Theo? Well…

He filled every part of her thoughts, both day and night. Or at least he had, until now. He still had no idea of her past or history. She still had no real desire to tell him. When he'd told her the other night that he had confidence in her when she was by his side at work, her heart had almost swollen to fill her chest.

Addy always managed to put on an outwardly positive appearance of confidence. But the real truth was all the dealings and deceptions with Stuart had stripped much of her confidence away. Things had all seemed as if they were slotting back into place—and now this.

She put down her fork, before she sent her body into overload. Her phone rang before she had a chance to think.

'Laura?' she asked.

The voice at the end of the phone was confused. 'No, it's Theo. Is everything okay?'

Heat flushed her cheeks. 'Yes, yes, everything's fine. What's wrong?'

She heard his deep breath. 'I hate to ask you

this, but the daycare have asked if I can go and pick up Max. He's running a temperature, but I have a patient requiring surgery for an implantable defibrillator in the next hour. I really don't want to cancel or delay.'

'It's fine,' she heard herself say without really thinking about it. 'I can collect Max.'

She heard a huge sigh of relief. 'Thanks. I wouldn't normally ask, but—'

'Where's the card for your apartment?' she asked. 'And do you have medicine I can give Max?'

'In my locker—the code is one, nine, six, seven—and, yes, I have kids' paracetamol and kids' ibuprofen. He's had them before with no problem and can take them alternately if running a temperature. I promise I'll be back in a few hours.'

'You'll be back when your patient is stable,' she cut in. 'Don't worry about Max. I can manage him for a few hours. If there's any problem I'll get a message to you.'

'I know,' he said, and there was a warmth in her skin.

He meant it. He trusted her. He trusted her with the most precious thing to him. She grabbed her light jacket and made her way to the hospital. It was literally only five minutes from the apartments. When she reached daycare, Theo had already phoned to say she was on her way.

The staff gave her a note with his temperature readings. He was flushed and sleepy when she picked him up. She'd never actually carried Max before, and three-year-olds were heavier than expected. But she heaved him up on one hip, and he tucked his arms around her neck as he sagged into her.

If he objected to her picking him up, he didn't say.

By the time she reached the apartment, he was like a leaden weight in her arms. She scanned open the door, carrying Max straight through to his bedroom.

She laid him on of the bright bed covers and took off his shoes. It only took her a moment to find the ear thermometer Theo had said he kept in his kitchen cupboard. Thirty-eight point five. High, but not enough to panic. She found the medicine, measured it out and propped him up a little, getting him take it along with a few sips of water.

All he wanted to do was sleep. And Addy knew the feeling well. On the few occasions she was sick, she just wanted to sleep too. The air conditioning in the apartment was on, and she made sure it was set at a level to keep him comfortable. She contemplated stripping off his T-shirt and shorts, but then settled on checking there was no obvious rash on his torso or back.

Children were always a worry. Infections, viruses, meningitis. She hadn't asked Theo if Max had been given his childhood vaccinations, but she was sure he wouldn't have left him at risk. She seemed to remember having to provide her own vaccination history for entry into Dubai as part of her visa requirements to stay and work here.

She wrote down Max's current temperature along with the time she'd given the medicine, and the amount, then settled in the chair in his room. It seemed wrong to sit in the other room. It didn't matter he was sleeping. She'd been asked to care for him, and she would.

She kept an eye on the clock and took his temperature half an hour later. It remained the same and she swithered about giving the other medicine. But another half an hour on it was at thirty-eight degrees. She gave Max a little shake and persuaded him to drink some more sips of water, before letting him sleep again.

She'd just walked through to the kitchen to look for something to drink herself when Theo came through the door.

It was clear he was worried, as he hurriedly said thanks and went straight through to Max's room. She wanted to walk after him, but decided to give him some time on his own. He came back, just as she was pouring some juice from a bottle in the fridge. He had the little note in his hand. Addy gave a shrug. 'The daycare had started it so I just kept it going. He'll be due his temp again in another five minutes.'

Theo ran his fingers through his hair.

'How's your patient?' she asked.

'Good,' he said as she handed the juice over to him and poured another glass for herself. 'Everything was straightforward, and they'll page me if there are problems overnight.'

She paused. 'Want me to stay?'

The words hung between them for a few seconds, as if they were both contemplating what that might mean. If, for some emergency, Theo did get called back to his patient, what would he do? If Max had already been sent home from daycare, they wouldn't accept him into the emergency overnight childcare at the hospital.

'That would be great,' he said. His eyes met hers, and she swallowed, trying to work out if it was just nerves, or something else.

It seemed like saying something without saying something. This would be the first time in a week she hadn't crept back to her own apartment in the early hours.

He went back through to check on Max again, took his temperature, wrote it down, then gave him the alternate medicine after getting him to drink a little more.

'Any idea what it is?' she asked.

He shook his head. 'Paediatrics was never my speciality. I've bought a Dr Spock book, another called *What's that Rash?* and joined an online group where people run symptoms past fellow parents.'

She folded her arms and looked at him in amusement. 'The kind of group that all health-care professionals cringe about?'

'Exactly that kind of group. And I like it,' he said, smiling as he waited for her barrage of abuse.

He opened his fridge and cringed. 'Not much here. We were planning on scrambled eggs on toast tonight, or pancakes and bacon.'

He looked at her expression and pulled out a plastic tub from the freezer. 'I'm better at this, honestly. I have pasta with five types of veg in it, bolognaise with hidden veg and lots of bases for homemade pizzas.'

She laughed. 'Dessert. What I really want is dessert.'

He went into the bottom tray of the freezer. 'Chocolate fudge cake, two minutes in the microwave and it's a dream.'

'Done,' she said rapidly.

A few minutes later they sat down at his dining table, spoons in hand. But Theo didn't start eating. He just sat for a few moments, fixing his gaze on the table.

She reached over and brushed her fingers against his. 'What?'

He blinked. 'What would I have done if you weren't here?'

He looked panicked. It had obviously played on his mind at points throughout the last few hours. 'You would have worked something out,' she said steadily.

'But what?' he persisted.

She held up her hand. 'They knew your circumstances when they took you on. Everyone gets sick kids. Your only option for childcare is the care they provide. They also know that. If Max is too sick for daycare, or the night option if you're on call, they have to provide cover.'

He ran his hands through his hair. She was starting to realise this was a sign of his nerves. 'For him, or for me?'

She stopped for a minute. It would make sense for them to provide a sitter if Max was sick. Because that would have to be less expensive than paying another doctor to cover Theo's shifts.

'Because I have no intention of leaving Max when he's sick, with someone that he and I don't know.'

It was reasonable. She knew it was reasonable.

And it was clear this was on his mind because he'd never been in this position before.

'Well, I guess you need to chat to someone about that.' She looked him in the eye. 'If I'm not working, and there's an issue with Max, then I'm happy to help, just like today. But if I'm working too, I'm not sure what the answer is.'

She was careful with her words. She didn't want to presume he would want her. She also needed to protect herself and her new role here. She couldn't pull a sickie because someone else's child was sick. And she hoped Theo would never ask her to. Was her job less important than his? It was a road she didn't want to go down.

The reason she was here, in this role in Dubai, was to support herself and get her head back above water. Lots of staff she knew had issues when their children were sick. It was a common problem—it was a fact of life that children tended to catch a myriad of minor ailments when they were young. While she was happy to assist when she could, she didn't want to become a crutch that Theo would expect was always available. Things were brand-new between them. It wasn't fair on either of them.

But, as she'd watched Max sleeping, his pale blond hair against the dark blue pillow, something in her heart had definitely pinged. Was this her biological clock finally telling her at thirty-two it was time to consider if children would be part of her future?

She'd watched other friends meet partners and have families, and it had never really featured in her head. It had always been in the place of *someday*, but it struck her today that the word *never* had not been one of the options she'd considered.

Of course, she didn't know if she could have children. Most people didn't until they started trying. There was nothing significant in her medical history. No past cancers along with invasive treatment…no gynaecological issues. But what if, with no opportunity of choice, she was already a no?

She hated these thoughts.

Theo looked worried, and tired again. Was he getting enough sleep?

'How about I sleep on the sofa?' she asked.

He blinked as if he hadn't had time to give her sleeping place much thought. She didn't want to suggest they sleep in the same room, particularly when Max was sick. Although Theo had said he always stayed in his own bed, Addy didn't want to bank on that.

'You can have my bed,' he said. 'I'll likely just sleep in the chair in Max's room. I want to keep checking his temp to make sure I keep on top of things.'

She wouldn't have expected any less. His fingers brushed against hers. 'Thanks, Addy. I really appreciate this.'

'No problem,' she said.

'And if I get called back to the hospital for any reason, I'll come and let you know before I go.'

She gave him a smile and a nod of her head. After another quick check on Max, she headed through to Theo's room. It wasn't a typical guy room. There were no dark colours. All his bedding was cream, but as soon she rested her head on the pillow she could smell him. The aftershave he wore, the scent of his skin, which was quickly becoming addictive.

I'm in trouble was the first thought in her head, rapidly followed with, *How truthful should I be?*

The letter and call to the solicitor had her worried. She knew she hadn't done anything wrong. She knew she'd been deceived by someone who'd likely done it before. It would be embarrassing enough to admit that to Theo, but what about the potential complications? The police might now suspect she wasn't innocent. They might want to charge her with something. That would put her job and work permit at risk. She hadn't declared any convictions because she didn't have any.

The last thing Theo would want is a potential criminal around his child. What if he didn't believe her?

Her stomach clenched and she wrapped her arms around herself as she lay in bed.

She was unsure about everything. Should this relationship continue? What if she got closer to Theo and Max, and then something happened that would make her have to return to Scotland? Max had already had a change in his life. How would Theo feel if the next woman he introduced Max to then disappeared from his life?

Her night was unsettled. Addy got up a few times, to check on both Theo and Max. Although Max was sometimes restless, his temperature didn't go any higher, and he slept for most of the night. He wasn't even surprised when Addy went in and spoke to him in the morning before she left for work.

Theo walked her to the door, giving her a hug and a kiss on the cheek. He gave a half-hearted smile. 'Sorry, we likely spoiled all your plans for last night.'

'I had no plans,' she said without hesitation, 'And I was happy to help.' She nodded over his shoulder. 'Will you be okay today?'

He nodded. 'I'm not scheduled to work today. I'll just have a lazy day watching Max and hopefully getting him on the road to recovery. Hopefully see you at work tomorrow.'

She gave a smile and headed out of the apartment and into her own. She blinked as she opened the front door and the brilliant sun met her, since none of her blinds were closed. What struck her most of all was the emptiness of the place, and the starkness of the décor.

She'd meant to get a few things to brighten the place up, but just hadn't got around to it yet. As she walked around, she realised she'd been here six weeks now, and the place didn't even look like her own.

Why was that? Her last flat had been full of her things—some of which she'd had to get rid of when she knew the place was being repossessed. Was that why she was reluctant to decorate? In case things got taken away from her again?

Addy sagged down on her own sofa. She was here for a fresh start. She'd met someone new. Things were looking good. She had to start focusing on the future—her future, and not the one that her toxic ex was trying to drag her into.

She looked around. It was time to put down some roots. Give herself something to fight for. Theo and Max were worth fighting for.

She was worth fighting for. She had to believe that.

CHAPTER NINE

THEO WAS GLAD that Max's temperature had settled and things appeared to be back to normal. He was a doctor, he should be able to handle a sick child, but the truth was it had caught him unawares.

It wasn't even the practical stuff—like having to find alternative childcare. It was the gut punch to the stomach that Max was sick. He couldn't really control it, and the fear of what if something actually happened to him?

He'd never been a parent. He'd never had a kid. This whole range of emotions had swept the feet out from under him. Theo had never had this responsibility before. It was all on him.

And he wasn't a fool. He'd known this when he'd taken on the future care of Max. But the emotional part had been overwhelming.

He doubted Addy even realised how much it meant to have another human around him at those moments. He was treading so carefully. They were only just together. The spark and passion between them was electrical. He was finding it hard to strike the right balance here—even though they'd spent every evening together for the last week. Tonight was the first time she'd stayed overnight—and Max hadn't even noticed. Theo was still finding his feet around being a parent. He couldn't expect her to take on his responsibilities alongside him. It wasn't fair to her, or to Max.

But a tiny part of him hoped for the future. Addison Bates was in his mind most days, and definitely every evening. A glimpse of her eyes, a flick of her hair, the sound of her laugh. Parts of him were being touched that he hadn't exposed in a long time.

If he could have sat down and planned a future, he wouldn't have met Addy yet. He would have settled in Dubai for a few years, cementing the relationship between him and Max. Then he would have got to know someone slowly, gradually introducing him to Max over months, before finally deciding to date.

But life had made its own plan for Theo. Maybe they'd already moved things too fast? But it was too late now, and he didn't have any regrets about her. She was a good person. He liked her straight-talking on the ward. She was kind to Max. She'd helped out without hesitation when he really needed it. She'd made something burn deep inside him that he hadn't even realised he needed. It was almost like he craved her, and that brought a smile to his face.

At work, they caught each other's eyes throughout the day like secret messages. There were definite secret smiles. But had anyone noticed yet? He didn't think so. They were still professional. But it was amazing what you could say to each other in an office on a ward that looked out on all the staff when the door was closed and they were at either end of the table. He just hoped no one could read lips.

She knew him, and she knew his life. But what did he really know about her? Not too much. Although she'd filled him in on the basics, he wanted to dig a little deeper. He wanted to know more, because he sensed there was still a barrier between them.

It was up to him to push a little further.

The staffing numbers on the ward had slowly got back up to normal. His workload had slightly increased because he and the other consultants were spreading Dr Gemmill's workload and patients between them.

It was fine. He still wasn't anywhere near as busy as he'd been in the general hospital back home in France.

The phone in the office rang and he answered it, talking to one of the Emergency physicians. He listened to the case. 'Fifteen-year-old, plays rugby, collapsed today on the pitch, was slightly cyanotic on the field. His ECG shows some unusual changes, his cardiac echo shows signs of apparent strain, and his chest X-ray also shows a slightly enlarged heart—but not significantly so. I know he's under eighteen, but this is a large kid, adult height and weight, and I wondered if you'd consider admitting him for cardiac review?'

Theo's decision was made in an instant. 'Have you taken bloods? Good, then add these tests to his panel and send him up. I'm happy to review his cardiac issues.'

He walked along the corridor until he found Addy. He gave her a smile. 'Charge Nurse Bates, as per our newly agreed admission protocol, I'd like to let you know about a fifteen-year-old we're admitting from Accident and Emergency after a collapse on a rugby field, and a number of unusual cardiac findings. Here's his details and the tests that have been run.' He handed her a slip of paper he'd taken notes on.

'Does he have a parent with him?'

Theo cringed. 'Oops. Forgot to ask.'

She shook her head. 'And that's why I'm the boss. If he took unwell at school, he might have come directly via the rugby pitch. I'll make enquiries to ensure his relatives are notified and are on their way.'

He leaned over and whispered in her ear. 'I'm

making dinner tonight. Singapore noodles. Do you prefer chicken or prawn?'

She took a quick glance sideways to see if anyone was listening. When she was assured their conversation was private she beamed at him. 'Both.'

He smiled. 'Both it is.'

By the time the patient came up from Emergency, his bloods were already available. Theo went directly into the room, wheeling a machine behind him so he could show the results to his patient.

'Khalid, I'm Dr Dubois. I'll be looking after you.'

Addy walked in behind him. 'Mum and Dad have just arrived downstairs and are on their way up.'

Theo sat down at the side of the bed. 'Tell me what happened today.'

Khalid was a fit-looking fifteen-year-old. He was as tall as Theo, had defined muscles and had obviously been playing rugby for a while.

Khalid put his hand to his chest. 'I don't really know. I was playing rugby, my legs started to feel heavy, my breathing hurt and then everything went black.'

'Any episodes like this before?'

Khalid frowned. 'I've been trying to get fitter. But instead of getting easier, I feel like things are getting worse. I don't have the same stamina. My running sprint times are going down, and I get out of breath easier.'

'Is this recent?'

'Fairly recent.' The boy gave a sigh. 'I go to the gym too, usually every day. I've been taking protein shakes.' He prodded at one bicep. 'My muscles are building okay, but I'm still overtired.' He looked annoyed. 'Other guys in my team can last much longer than I can.'

There was a noise behind Theo, and he turned to see the anxious faces of Khalid's parents, who'd obviously heard some of what had been said.

His mum rushed over and put her hand on her son's head. 'Are you okay? They told me you'd collapsed.'

'What's wrong with him?' Khalid's dad directed the question to Theo.

Theo held out his hand. 'Dr Dubois. I'm a cardiologist and I'm looking after your son.'

'A cardiologist? Something's wrong with his heart?' Worry creased their faces, as well as Khalid's.

Theo held up one hand. 'Accident and Emergency have asked me to review Khalid. They ran a number of standard tests when he came in that I'm just about to check over. One of the things that was reported was that Khalid's lips were blue—we call it cyanotic—when he took unwell. Since he has no history of asthma or lung problems, and his temperature was entirely normal, because his lips are blue, the next thing we check is the heart.'

He wasn't sure he'd relieved any of their stress, but at least they all looked as if they understood. He faced both parents. 'I was asking Khalid about his fitness and he's telling me he's been feeling more tired than he thinks he should. Have you noticed anything that worries you?'

His dad held his hand towards the bed. 'Well, he's a teenager. They're meant to sleep a lot, aren't they?'

Khalid's mum wrinkled her nose. 'I guess he does seem more tired than usual. He started rugby in the last two years and he's been doing really well. But he's lost his spark in the last while.' She grimaced as she said the words, knowing that her son was overhearing her.

But Theo just nodded, taking in all the information. He'd already had a look at the test results, and Khalid was currently attached to a heart monitor and blood pressure cuff.

'Has your son been unwell at all in the last year?'

There were some exchanged glances. Finally, the mum shrugged. 'He had a bit of a fever more than a month ago, a rash, and his tongue was red and swollen. We were told he'd had a possible allergic reaction to something. But we never understood what. It's probably been since then that he hasn't really got back to normal.'

Theo swallowed, his mind instantly going to a place that could explain what the tests showed, and the boy's current symptoms. It wasn't good.

'Okay. Exactly how long ago was this?'

The mum pulled out her phone. 'It was when we were invited to a family dinner. Khalid didn't come as he couldn't eat much. Here,' she turned her phone around, 'just over six weeks ago.'

Addy moved across the room and put a hand on his shoulder. She knew where this conversation would go.

Theo spun the monitor around so Khalid and his parents could see it. 'Okay, this is a scan of Khalid's heart. See these parts?' He pointed to particular sections. 'This is part of the heart muscle, and it looks as if it's under strain. You can see it here, and here. It's thicker than normal, meaning the heart is having to work harder to circulate the blood.'

He pulled up Khalid's ECG. 'I know this just looks like squiggles, but it tells me quite a lot. It also says that Khalid's heart is showing signs of strain.'

'He's never had heart problems,' said the dad quickly.

Theo gave a nod to indicate that he'd heard. 'I

also looked at the blood tests. They show signs of inflammation in Khalid's body.'

Theo took a breath. 'From the previous symptoms you've told me about, and how Khalid is now, I think the event six weeks ago wasn't an allergic reaction. I think Khalid had Kawasaki disease.'

'What's that?' asked the mum.

'The diagnosis is unusual,' said Theo steadily, 'it usually shows in children under six, but can be diagnosed in young adults. It sounds as if it was missed.'

'So, you can fix it?' asked the dad. 'Give him something?'

Theo kept his voice calm. 'Kawasaki disease is an inflammatory disease that affects the blood vessels and heart. If it's picked up early, there are treatment options, and we will look at some medicines for Khalid. But if it's missed—Khalid's was—there can be long-term effects.' He turned to face Khalid. 'Some of the symptoms you have today make me think there could be damage to your heart and surrounding blood vessels. This can also happen to children who are diagnosed quickly and given treatment.'

'Where does this come from? Did he catch it from someone?'

Theo shook his head. 'No one really knows the cause as yet. Some researchers think it's the body's own response to an infection, some think that certain genetic factors predispose people to the condition. There's also been research into environmental factors, but nothing definitive has been found.'

Khalid put his hands to his chest. 'Am I going to die?'

It was the hardest question to answer. Because the real truth was, he just didn't know. Depending on the damage the disease had caused, Khalid could be at risk.

'We need to find out how your systems have been affected, and then we look at how we can monitor or minimise any damage that's been done. I'm going to start you on a really simple drug called aspirin straightaway, because it's good at preventing any clots forming.'

'What about my rugby, and the gym?'

This time Addy stepped in as she moved to the side of Khalid's bed. 'The doctors need to get as much information as possible right now. Once they have it all, they'll be able to let you know about future plans.'

Theo turned to the parents. 'We'll run some more tests, but I'd like to refer Khalid to a specialist I know. He's actually a paediatric cardiologist in another city. Although Khalid is almost an adult, this disease usually presents in children younger than Khalid, and this paediatrician is an expert in people with this disease and their ongoing care. Are you happy for me to do that?'

Both parents nodded and Addy handed over some literature she'd printed off for them on the disease and its treatments.

They excused themselves and went to decide on more tests.

Once they hit the office, Addy turned to face him. 'Do you think he could have an aneurysm?' It was a known consequence of the disease.

'I'm praying he doesn't, but we'll run the tests anyway. From his symptoms I'm guessing he already has some narrowing of the arteries and could be at risk of an MI.'

Addy shuddered. 'A possible MI at fifteen? Please, no.'

She turned to her computer and pulled up the records. 'Did anyone see Khalid when he was unwell? This shouldn't have been missed.'

'I'll need to dig deeper,' he said. 'Someone must have seen him to suggest an allergic reaction. Or they may just have searched for "swollen tongue" online? In any case, if we find out Khalid was seen somewhere, we might need to suggest some training.'

'It's unusual at this age,' said Addy in a more conciliatory tone. 'I remember seeing a research article on the diagnosis of a twenty-one-year-old. That seemed old.'

'It is.' Theo nodded in agreement. 'But the long-term issues are just too great to ignore. If we find out this was missed, we need to take steps to make sure it doesn't happen again.' He'd finished writing up the rest of the tests that needed to be done, one of which was an angiogram to see if the coronary arteries were damaged.

'This poor kid,' said Addy. He could tell from her expression that she was worried about him. 'What if we have to tell him that rugby and the gym won't be on the cards for a while?'

'I'm hoping my colleague Brin Edson will be able to help with this one. He really is an expert, and even with risk factors involved he wants to keep these kids as healthy as possible and living their lives the best possible way.'

'Will he be able to see Khalid? You said he lives in another city?'

Theo nodded. 'Berlin. But we have the internet now—tests can be ordered, results sent and online consultations arranged. He's the best, and that's what Khalid should have. These are unique circumstances.'

'They are,' she agreed, then gave him a soft smile. 'Thank goodness you were working today.'

He shrugged. 'I'm sure one of the other cardiologists would have caught this.'

'But would they have known where to refer?'

'Maybe not, but we're a team. If someone had

told me about this case, I would advise them to consult Brin. I know about him because I attended a number of international conferences he's spoken at. This could just as easily have been another lesser-known condition, and maybe one of them would have pointed me in the right direction. We're all here to help each other and find the best thing for our patients.'

'Did anyone tell Dr Gemmill?' she joked.

He leaned back and then raised his eyebrows. 'You earned a clean sweep at the governance committee. You must be pleased. Everyone agreed with the suggestions and accepted the paper with no concerns.'

'That's only because Dr Gemmill is still off,' she replied, still smiling.

'Well, it doesn't matter what he thinks if he comes back,' said Theo. 'Because it's been agreed through all the processes. He'll need to follow them like everyone else.'

'It won't get me moved back to his ward though,' said Addy, her expression sad.

'Why would you want to go back there…' he held up his hands '…when you can work here with me?'

Her eyes gleamed and she gave him a wicked smile. 'Well, of course, I wouldn't. But…' She paused for a second. 'It still feels like I got hounded out of there, because I dared to question some of the practices.'

'Would you do anything different?'

She pressed her lips together. 'Probably not. It's unlikely he would have listened even if I'd spoken to him.' She held up one hand. 'I may have decided to speak to his secretary, but that wouldn't have solved the root of the problem.' Her gaze met Theo's. 'So, no. I wouldn't do anything different.'

'And that's why I like you,' he said.

She raised her eyebrows across the table at him.

He continued. 'Because you're stubborn, determined, and at the bottom of it all is good patient care, so who can argue with that?'

She leaned across the table towards him. 'Is that the only reason you like me? Or...' she smiled at him suggestively '...is it also because we share a love of desserts?' She winked. 'And a few other things?'

He laughed. He'd held his breath for a second, wondering what she might say.

'Come to think of it, you haven't mentioned dessert for tonight. You better remember to put that in the plans too.'

He rolled his eyes. 'Don't worry, I won't forget about dessert.' Then he stopped and looked at her again. 'What are your plans for the weekend?'

She shrugged. 'Not much. Shopping. The cream walls and furnishings are closing in around me. I need some colour in the place. I meant to get some things the other week, but time just got away from me.'

'What kind of shopper are you?'

'What do you mean?'

'Are you a mall girl? Or would you be willing to look in some of the markets and souks?'

She didn't hesitate for a second. 'Millionaire malls? No thanks. But I'm not sure where any of the markets are yet. I've not had a real chance to look around.'

'If you don't mind a few tag-alongs, Max and I will be happy to show you the markets and the souks at the weekend. I think you might find things that you like.'

She smiled. 'A weekend with my two favourite guys. Sounds like a plan.'

He leaned forward and sighed, putting his head in his hand. 'Honestly. You're too easy to charm. I haven't even told you my ulterior motive yet.'

Something fleeting passed her eyes and he saw her tense for a second, but then it disappeared. 'Dr Dubois, what is your ulterior motive?'

He gave a broad smile. 'It involves someone aged three. A very dark room. And the millionth movie about little yellow characters.' He raised his eyebrows. 'I might even try to touch your leg in the dark.'

She laughed. 'You want to go to the pictures?'

'The what?'

She grinned. 'The pictures. That's what we call the cinema in Scotland.'

He frowned and shook his head. 'So, you call going to see a film or a movie "the pictures"?'

'Of course, and so should everybody else—it would save a whole lot of hassle.'

He loved that, when her Scottish accent came through thicker than before and he had to concentrate on her words.

'So, will you come?'

'Is there popcorn?'

'There is.'

She leaned forward. 'Then I'll come.' Then she whispered, 'And just between you and me, I kind of like those yellow creatures.'

A warm feeling spread through him. He was almost sure other staff in the department had started to talk about them. But honestly? He didn't care. As long as this relationship didn't affect their work, it was no one else's business.

Relationship? Had he thought about it in those terms before? No, because he wasn't quite sure what to call it. Using the word relationship might be presumptuous.

But it didn't feel like that to him. In fact, as the word settled in his brain, it felt quite comfortable. He was happy around Addy. After their prickly start, he'd liked her almost immediately. She was easy to like.

And she was making an impact at work. Staff had started to realise just how scarily organised she was. She had spreadsheets for costs, rotas and some baseline information on average stays on the ward.

She'd set some staff the task of reviewing the wards' standard operating procedures, and preparing some new ones for tasks that hadn't quite made it to that stage yet. This was a teaching hospital, and it was good to have a start-to-finish plan for some procedures to show students before they accompanied staff on their rounds. It helped their learning and gave them a good minimum baseline.

The idea around staff rotating was also taking wings. Apparently, some staff had asked in the past and been turned down, but with Addison's backing, the planning processes were now in place, and it looked like it would be starting soon.

Her organisation and leadership were being noticed in the space of a few short months. Now Dr Gemmill wasn't around, he heard more of the consultants saying how good she was. She'd assisted in Theatre more than once during the sickness period, and had also taken charge of a night shift in the cardiac ICU after a member of staff had a sudden family bereavement.

People were seeing Addison for who she truly was. And it wasn't just staff and management. Feedback from patients was good too. Her bedside manner was straightforward but fun. She encouraged questions and had the patience to take her time explaining things at a level patients understood.

He'd heard on the grapevine that she'd been invited on a few staff night outs and turned them down. But she had joined the local hospital book group and was apparently a vociferous reader.

But the most important thing to Theo was how things were between them. She was good to Max. She didn't mind teasing or flirting with Theo as long as no one else was around, and the buzz he got when she looked at him with those violet eyes…

It was the first time in a long time that he was considering something more serious. He couldn't deny the attraction, or the feelings he had for Addison. They'd naturally fallen into a pattern of spending every evening together. Maybe it was time to have a conversation about being official? Letting others know they were actually in a relationship? Maybe this weekend would be the right time?

He could swear he almost felt a fizzing in his

belly. But he wanted to do this. He wanted to have the grown-up conversation. They had a connection that neither of them could ignore, and which they continued to act on, most nights when Max was in bed. He knew how she took her coffee. What biscuits were her favourite. What she preferred to watch on TV. Which old-school nineties band was her secret favourite. And knowing all of these things sent a warm glow around him. One that he wanted to continue, to grow and develop. He smiled to himself. Could little yellow characters assist him? He'd have to wait and find out.

'I would never have found this place,' said Addy as she looked from side to side underneath her wide-brimmed hat.

The market was buzzing, stalls and small stores everywhere. There was a huge array of wonderful smells. The constant background noise of voices and shouts of laughter was pleasant and welcoming. But the thing that captured her attention most was the bursts of colour.

Furniture, clothing on people, clothing for sale. Items for houses in a wide range of hues. She was trying to pretend she couldn't see all the gold that was available for barter, as she wasn't there to spend vast amounts of money. She wasn't sure she would ever be in a position to do that again. But rugs, vases, cushions and prints…they were all on her mind to bring some colour into her apartment and make it feel more like home.

They threaded themselves through the bustling crowd. Max was fascinated, stopping to stare at things, asking multiple questions and being taken in by all the street vendors around the sides.

They moved into a bigger area and Addy's eyes were caught by a giant sofa. It was in the window of one of the stores and was covered like patchwork in a bright array of fabrics. She'd seen similar designs in some magazines in the past—all with spectacular price tags.

'Wow,' was all she could say.

Theo followed her over and grinned. 'Now, that's perfect.'

'You think?' she asked, eyes full of excitement.

'It's my dream. If I spilled something on that, you'd never know.'

She nudged him in the side and groaned but he grabbed her hand and pulled her inside.

'Let's try it,' he said, pulling Max up onto his knee as he sat and Addy down beside him. The giant sofa gave a *hmph* noise as they all sat down, making them burst out with laughter.

Addy ran her hand over the array of fabric. Some velvet, some heavy stitching, some linen, some felt more like a rug. But the colours were like an explosion—reds, yellows, oranges, browns, the odd patch of purple or green. It was like a whole story being told beneath her eyes. And the padding was just luxurious.

She looked out through the store window and realised people were looking in on them. It made her laugh out loud. She ran her hand across the fabrics again, then moved it down to the wooden claw foot. It might not be to everyone's taste, but she loved it.

'Well, this would certainly give you a burst of colour in the apartment. You wouldn't need anything else.'

She rested her head backward. 'If only.'

'I like it,' said Max.

'So do I,' said Theo. 'But Addy spotted it first.'

She gave a sigh and stood up. 'This will be well outside my price range. Come on, guys, I need to find a vase and some cushions.'

Her hand trailed across the back where the price tag was. Feeling just a little curious she flicked it over. Her gulp was a kind of semi-gulp. It wasn't as pricey as she feared, but the little savings she had in the bank she needed to keep. If the solicitor phoned to say the police were demanding she return at short notice, she'd need money for flights, and somewhere to stay for a few days.

Theo was by her side, looking at the tag. 'Well, that's okay,' he said, his brown eyes connecting with hers. 'Are you going to get it?'

Spoken like a man who'd never had his house

repossessed or had to account for everything he spent.

She couldn't help it. It made her ultra-defensive. 'Not in my price range,' she said quickly. 'Let's just get the things that are.'

As soon as the words were out of her mouth, she wanted to kick herself. This was definitely a conversation she didn't want to have.

'Okay,' Theo said quietly behind her, but she could hear the question in his voice and it made all her senses go on alert. Theo had never mentioned money. As far as she knew, he didn't have any money concerns. His biggest issue had been childcare, and he'd solved that by taking the job in Dubai.

Hoping he was following her, she moved quickly to a stall with brightly coloured vases, picking a medium-sized one decorated in merged swirls of pink and red. Then she chose two cushions with red backgrounds, and a bright tablecloth for the table just outside her kitchen.

By the time she'd finished, Max was back by her side eating some small sweets. Theo held out a bag. 'Want some?'

She shook her head, feeling awkward and a bit foolish. 'I'm done, I've got everything I need. These should brighten my apartment up a bit.'

'Shall we head back?' he asked. 'We'll need to

drop those things off before we go…' He hesitated, and then added, 'To the pictures.'

He said the words in the worst Scottish accent ever and she couldn't help but laugh. 'Okay then, give me a hand.' She handed the vase over to him and they travelled back to the apartment to drop off her purchases.

Even as she glanced around the space, there was a little knot in her stomach. The patchwork sofa would have been more than perfect for this place. It would have drawn the eye straight away and sent a message of warmth, happiness and welcome. It stung her so bad, her breath caught somewhere in her throat.

She blinked back the tears that threatened to fall and walked her vase over to her side table. It was lovely. The cushions on her sofa were good too, and the tablecloth on the dining table just outside the kitchen tied everything together.

Her apartment was coming together—just like her relationship with Max and Theo. There was a constant flutter around her heart and buzz around her stomach. Everything felt too good and too soon. And, the trouble was, Theo had no idea that the tower they were magically building together was actually teetering. Another letter from the police or phone call from her solicitor could bring this perfect world she'd accidentally created crashing down around her.

And what she knew above all else was that she really, really didn't want that to happen. She took a deep breath and fixed a smile on her face.

'Better than I could have hoped for,' she said quickly to Theo and Max, who were patiently waiting for her, and she ignored that knot again. 'Let's go and meet my favourite little yellow people.' She grabbed her bag and held her hand out to Max. He threaded his hand into hers with an innocence that made her catch her breath, and then she headed back out into the Dubai sunshine with them.

Theo wasn't entirely sure what he'd done wrong. But from the look on her face, and the snap of her words, he'd suddenly realised that money must be an issue for Addison.

It was easy to forget these things when their accommodation came as part of the employment deal—lots of staff stayed in these luxury apartments. Maybe she had family issues and had to send a large part of her salary home. One of the doctors that he worked with had told him freely that he sent more than half his salary home to support his mum, dad and disabled sister. Not all countries had free health care available or government assistance for those unable to work.

That was the trouble. He still didn't know her

well enough. But that wasn't stopping the flood of feelings he was getting caught up in.

He had to try and get her to trust him. To talk to him more. Because he wanted this to work. He was more invested than ever.

Every time she walked into his apartment his heart seemed to lift a little. Each time he watched her effortlessly interact with Max it sent a warm sensation through his veins. He might not have been ready. But it looked like the world had other plans for him.

He'd bought the tickets for the cinema online. As soon as Max saw the posters with his favourite yellow characters he started bouncing up and down on his toes. It only took Theo a few moments to buy them popcorn before they were filing their way into the dimmed cinema.

Max sat between them to begin with. Then changed seats partway through the film because he had to go to the bathroom. By the time Theo sat down next to Addy, he could tell she'd started to relax again.

When they finally left the cinema, he reached out as they exited the row, and she took his hand.

They travelled back on the Dubai Metro and, when he suggested picking up takeout on the way back, she was happy to agree.

Max was wilting—the fun of the market, then concentrating in the cinema had all got too much for him. Theo carried him the last few yards to the apartment block, and laid him down on his bed when they got home.

Instead of sitting at the table, they kept their takeout in the boxes and sat on the sofa together, with cans of soda on the floor next to them.

Once they'd started eating, Theo decided to dig a little deeper.

'So, what about Scotland? Are you planning on going back, or will you stay here now?'

She gave a half-shrug. 'I haven't made any decisions yet. I wasn't sure how things would go here, or if I'd like it.'

'And do you like it?' he asked, with a gleam in his eye.

He watched her for a second, and as he waited he had a flash of fear that her answer might actually be no. But she let out a little sigh, her shoulders relaxed. As her gaze met his she said, 'Better than I thought I would.'

He smiled and then gave her a slow nod. 'It's tough going somewhere new where you don't know anyone. Because of the circumstances I'm in, it's not like I can meet new people and go out for a beer together.'

'Your fellow consultants would go out for a beer?' She raised her eyebrows, clearly in disbelief.

He laughed. 'The rest of the cardiologists are

a bit older than me. But there's some surgeons my age, a couple of anaesthetists, and a group of physios that have started a football team. If I was here on my own, that's the kind of thing I might do.'

She looked at him for a moment. 'But, if you were on your own, you wouldn't have come here, would you?'

He shook his head. 'No, you're right, I wouldn't have.' He took a slow breath. 'Things are exactly the way they should be.'

Her nose wrinkled just a little. 'So, you never get angry at Fleur? You never wonder why she couldn't beat her addiction for Max, or maybe have let you know who his father was, so he could have played a part in their life?'

The question troubled him, but only because the answer wasn't too nice. 'I did get angry at Fleur—lots of times. That's part of why I pushed her into making a will. But Fleur was an adult. And she'd been my friend, but I wasn't responsible for her. I'm not an expert on addiction, but I, and the rest of her friends and family, tried to support her. But addicts frequently push people away. I'm pretty sure Max's father was an addict too, and I know that, although she'd reduced her use during her pregnancy, Max still had to go through a withdrawal regime after he was born.' He put his hand to his chest. 'And honestly, that

made me furious, that she'd done that to her baby.
But I didn't doubt she loved him. When I watched
them together, there was genuine love and affection between them. She just loved her addiction
more.'

Addison shuddered. 'That's terrifying.'

He looked at her expression. 'It is, but it's not
unique. My biggest worry for Max is the stuff I
don't know about.'

'What do you mean?'

It struck him for a moment that this was not
where he wanted this conversation to go. He
wanted to learn more about *her*. But things had
kind of got turned around, and the truth was,
Addy was so easy to talk to.

He sighed. 'The research about kids says their
first few years are the most formative. I have no
idea what Max's day-to-day experience was. I
hope it was good. But I know that sometimes
Fleur would have been using drugs, and I wonder if he remembers being ignored or neglected.'

Her hand reached over and slid into his. 'You
have no way of knowing that. And I get what you
say, but you're assuming the worst. You know that
she loved Max. Didn't she?'

He nodded. 'But her addiction was real. It took
over parts of her life.'

'Did you meet many of her friends then?'

He wrinkled his brow. 'Sometimes. Most were

fleeting, in and out of her life, dealing with their own issues.'

'But…' She was clearly taking her time with this answer. 'They may also have helped her when she needed it. Maybe if she was having a bad spell, one or other of those folks would have looked out for Max. He's a sweet kid. Pretty adorable.'

She was trying to be reassuring, and he admired her for it, recognising this was a line of conversation that could never come to a definitive conclusion.

'I hope so,' he said. 'I hope that's what happened.'

There was silence for a moment before he met her violet gaze again.

'You didn't really mention what made you leave Scotland.' He knew he was pushing. But it felt like it was time.

She started with the normal words. 'Opportunity, better money, a new start.' But as her words tailed off, they both realised this was the expected answer, not the actual truth.

He kept his voice steady. 'You know that this is building to something, don't you?'

She gave the briefest nod of her head.

'And Max has become my world.'

She nodded again.

He ran his fingers through his hair. 'So, I've

met someone, unexpectedly, that I really like.' He locked gazes with her. '*More* than like.'

She held that gaze and he continued. 'And I hope…' His heart gave a little flutter. This could be the moment he made the biggest fool of himself on the planet. 'That she likes me too. Likes *us* too.'

Addy seemed as though she were frozen in place.

He kept going, hoping he wasn't about to wreck things between them. 'So, I realised that I don't know that much about her—that much about you. And I wondered if there was anything you needed to tell me?'

Her head had lowered but now whipped fiercely up. 'What, you think I'm some kind of criminal?'

He jerked back as if stung, wondering why that had been the first place she'd gone. He held up one hand. 'No, not at all. You just haven't said much about your family, or your friends, or anything about past relationships, and I just thought I should ask.'

Her eyes looked fierce now. 'Did it ever occur to you that if people don't talk about something there's a reason for that?'

His stomach was cringing. 'Of course, I know that. But the more time I spend with you, the more I want to know about you. Is that wrong?'

But the words didn't seem to placate her. It was

clear that all her red flags had gone up around him. 'So, you think I'm a risk?'

He shook his head again. 'No, no, it's just that—'

He didn't get to finish as she cut him off. 'So, you *do* think I'm a risk.' It wasn't a question, it was a statement. Since when did trying to get to know someone a bit better set off this kind of response?

He could keep trying to placate her, or he could just cut right to the chase. 'I'm trusting you, Addy. I'm trusting you with being around Max, and sometimes being alone with him. And I do trust you. But you've also heard me tell you how much I worry about him. If I'd thought about this more, I maybe wouldn't have introduced you both so quickly. Five months ago he lost the central female in his life. Now I've let someone else in. And I've done it because I wanted to. It felt right. It felt good. But I have some questions. Are you telling me I shouldn't ask?'

She stood up. 'Frame it however suits you. But some parts of people's lives are private. We are all entitled to privacy, Theo. I don't need to tell you all my personal friendships or relationship disasters. That's for me to know. Not you.' She took a few steps. 'You know that Spira will have done a whole host of checks on me—like they did with you—before I started here. If there was anything significant, they wouldn't have offered me the job. What more do you need? My medical history? My family genetics?'

He stood up too. 'Whoa. This is getting way off track.'

'Is it?' He could see the anguish on her face, and immediately wondered why he'd let this reach this point. It never should have. But that deeply protective instinct in him was going wild. At the heart of this was a little boy. He'd just revealed his own vulnerabilities around his fears for Max. He couldn't say for sure, but he didn't think he was being unreasonable. He'd clearly hit a nerve with Addy—and he absolutely hadn't meant to. But his father-bear instincts were roaring loud and strong. He couldn't just think about himself any more. He and Max were a partnership, and he always had to take Max into consideration.

He lowered his voice. 'Addy, I'm just asking you if there's anything I need to know. If you're in trouble in any way, I'd like to help you.'

'I've never asked for your help,' she spat back.

Theo's shoulders sagged. While they were both on edge, this would never get anywhere helpful. He knew that, and he sensed she did too.

She walked over to the door. 'Thanks for the nice day,' she said, 'but I'm going to go home now.'

And before he had a chance to say anything else, she was gone.

* * *

Addy was furious. A fury that she couldn't contain, or really explain. In the few steps she'd taken down the corridor, hot, angry tears had spilled down her cheeks.

By the time she'd fumbled with her key card and got inside, her shoulders had started to go too.

The bright cushions, vase and tablecloth were like a gut punch now. She'd bought them to bring hope, joy and welcome vibes to her bare apartment. But they practically screamed Theo's and Max's names at her. This wasn't how this was supposed to go.

The phone in her apartment was blinking. She couldn't remember it ever doing that before, and she pressed the button to listen to the message.

And then the day just got worse.

'Hi, Addy, it's Laura Palmer here. I've spoken at length to the new inspector in charge of the case. It seems Stuart King has been laying on his charm quite heavily and appears to have almost convinced this man that some of the responsibility lies at your door. I've asked him to investigate digitally around IP addresses, for the loan agreements and signatures. I already know that one of the loans that was digitally signed was agreed on a date you were working a twelve-hour shift in Glasgow. However, he wants to reinterview you regarding the whole fraud episode. He initially insisted on an in-person interview, but I've persuaded him that would be unreasonable due to costs. He's agreed to a video interview, but we have to arrange a day and time. Can you get back to me when you get this message, please?'

Addy felt her legs go from under her. Her head was spinning. She'd already given an array of statements around Stuart's fraudulent activities. What else could they want?

Something flicked in her brain and it was like her blood had suddenly run cold. It had been a throwaway comment. Theo had likely meant nothing by it. But when he'd arranged this day together, he'd remarked she was too easy to charm.

What did that actually mean? Was she a fool? She thought she knew everything about him—but what if he'd been untruthful? What if, right now, Addison was being played, just like she'd been with Stuart? Hadn't she learned anything from that whole experience?

Her whole body was trembling now as she slid to the floor.

Was she misjudging everything?

She tried to calm herself and take some deep breaths. Things were just overwhelming her. The pressure of the mess she'd been left in back in Glasgow had been too much to cope with. She'd always been methodical and organised. To know that someone she'd loved had played her, had outsmarted her—it had made her question everything she thought she knew. The way that he'd also created doubts about her amongst their friend group had been the most hurtful aspect of all. For the first time in her life, all the fight had gone out of her. Once she'd finished with the police—when she knew the full extent of the accumulated debt and her flat repossession—she just wanted to get away.

The contact from her lawyer had taken her back to square one.

Her heart rate started to slow, and her breathing eased.

Theo Dubois wasn't Stuart King. He was a good guy. An honest one. But she still didn't want to share all this with him. Shopping today had freaked her out. The sofa had been gorgeous, and she would have loved it. But if she'd tried to purchase it, he might have thought it odd that she didn't have a credit card, and that wasn't a conversation she wanted to have.

A relationship had been the furthest thing from her mind when she'd come here. But it was almost like someone had landed Theo and Max on her lap. It felt fated—meant to be—and right now there was a chance she was going to blow everything.

What must he think of her?

Her experience with Stuart was clouding her

emotions and making her overthink things. Not every guy she met would be some kind of con man. She'd been unlucky. She knew that. But she had to try and move on.

She looked up at her phone on the table. If she really wanted to move on, she had to put everything behind her. And right now that would include talking to the police again. It didn't matter that she didn't want to relive any of this. Stuart was clearly up to something again, and was likely trying to clear his path to the next con.

She put her hand to her heart. He'd ruined her faith in herself, and her ability to trust. But that wasn't Theo's or Max's fault. She had to judge them on their own merits, no matter how hard she was finding things.

As she held her hand at her heart, she realised something. She loved them. She loved them both as a package deal—because that's what they would always be. It had sneaked up on her. But she had to acknowledge her true feelings. She was far too afraid to say those words out loud, but she couldn't help the wealth of emotions that were buried deep. Maybe that's why she was reacting so badly to things? Admitting that she loved them could change everything, and the world was spinning too quickly as it was.

She bent forward and let her head rest on her knees. Theo had already told her he 'more than liked her'. What would he think of her reaction today?

It must have shocked and surprised him. She could feel embarrassment sweep over her and more tears came to her eyes. She was so unsure about herself right now.

But the one thing she was absolutely sure about was that she wouldn't let Stuart King impact on her life any more. He'd destroyed the life she had back in Glasgow, and he wouldn't destroy the one she had here.

She did have to speak to Theo. She did need to tell him the truth about her past. But she wanted to do it on her own terms. She wanted to do it when she'd sorted things, so she could look him in the eye, be truthful and let him know she was out through the other side.

Then she would be ready to dive into this relationship with her eyes and arms wide open.

CHAPTER TEN

THEO WASN'T QUITE sure what had happened. One minute they were having a nice day together and the next… It still baffled him.

Had he misjudged everything? Maybe he'd misinterpreted her level of interest in him. Had he pushed her too far, too fast? He couldn't help the feelings of shock and disappointment he'd had around her reaction. There was nothing like telling someone he cared deeply about that he more than liked them, only to witness them pick a fight and almost sprint for the horizon.

Everything felt so terribly wrong. Maybe this was all his fault? Maybe he should have kept things going in their own easy way, without hinting at more, or a deeper connection. It was clear that Addy wasn't ready. Or at least wasn't ready for any more with him.

That made him sadder than he'd ever expected. He didn't just 'more than like' Addy. He loved her. But there was no chance to say that, and it seemed like the last thing she might want to hear.

For the next week they tiptoed around each other at work and in the apartment block. No real conversations. No real connection again.

Max kept asking if they could visit, or if Addy would visit them. Then he stayed mysteriously quiet about her. And that set off a whole lot of other worries that he'd let his little boy form an attachment with someone who might not really care about him.

But then there were a couple of texts out of the blue. The first was from Addy.

Was planning to drop into daycare to see Max. Is that okay with you?

He didn't answer straight away because he was momentarily stunned. Part of him wanted to jump in the elevator and go down there too. Maybe they could actually talk?

But something told him not to. This was about Max, not him. What was best for Max? His brain spun round and round.

One of the nurses came and asked him to pre-scribe something, so he texted back quickly.

Fine.

But when he went to pick up Max later, he never mentioned a word about Addy coming to see him. It was strange—and not like Max at all.

He waited a few moments before talking quietly to one of the staff members. 'I know Addy came down to see Max earlier but he hasn't mentioned her. Do you know if she told Max not to say anything?' he'd asked.

Doria, one of the staff, shook her head straightaway. 'I was playing alongside Addy and Max with another little boy. She never said anything like that at all to him.' Doria then pressed her lips together in sympathy. 'Maybe Max is picking up on something. Can you think of a reason he wouldn't tell you? He's kind of young to make that decision.'

But Theo knew exactly why Max wouldn't say anything, because he'd been in the room when Theo and Addy had exchanged words. It made his heart ache to think of the impact he was having on his son—because that was how he thought of Max now.

Max had likely suffered enough trauma in his life. The last thing he needed was any more. Theo's job was to make him feel safe and secure, and if his son wasn't telling him something, he needed to ask himself why.

The next day on the ward he walked into the office where Addy was sitting and closed the door behind him. She looked up in surprise.

'Is something wrong?' Although they'd worked together this last week, she'd barely met his eyes.

She'd just kept everything professional, with no real discussion.

'Yes,' he said bluntly, sitting down.

'What?'

'Max hasn't told me that you've been to see him at daycare.'

There was an awkward pause between them and Addy's brow furrowed. 'Okay,' she said slowly.

'That seems…strange.'

'I agree.'

'Why did you go to see him?' The question came out blunter than he meant.

She licked her lips slowly. 'I missed him, and I wanted to make sure he was doing okay.'

'You could have asked me how he was doing.'

She let out a long, slow breath. 'I could have, but it wouldn't be the same.'

He could swear a hand squeezed around his heart. Asking if someone was okay and seeing for yourself was entirely different. He appreciated that.

What also struck him was the fact that, when he'd challenged her on it, she was straight. She wasn't sorry at all that she'd seen Max.

And he knew. He knew how she felt.

'I don't want my son keeping secrets from me.'

She took a deep breath. 'I didn't ask him to.'

'I know.'

Tears pricked her eyes. 'So, where does that leave us?'

There was silence for a few moments before he added, 'I miss you, Addy. *We* miss you.'

'I miss you both too.' She put her head in her hands. 'I know this is my fault. I know it is.' She bit her lip. 'I have no right to ask, but could you just be a little patient with me please? I have a few things I need to sort out.'

Silence hung in the air between them while he turned things over in his mind. He knew better than to push again. So he didn't ask for details.

He spoke in a low voice. 'I don't want my little boy to get hurt. He's fond of you, Addy, you know he is.'

The tears spilled down her cheeks. 'And I'm fond of him too. I want to be around him. I want to be around you both.'

Theo let it hang a little longer, and then finally said, 'So, how do we fix this?'

She gave a huge sigh of relief. 'How about we all just take breath, and spend some time together again?' She put a hand on her heart. 'I promise, from my end, I will fix this.'

He smiled and moved around the table towards her. He wasn't going to push her again. He had to make the decision to take her on trust. Because he did want to spend time with her again, and he knew Max did too. 'What do you have in mind?'

'We could do a movie night at mine, or we could take Max swimming. I saw some lessons advertised and thought it might be good for him to start.'

Theo sat back and looked at her. He was impressed. 'I kept meaning to look for some.'

'Well, I've found them. Want me to set it up? We could go in after his lesson and get him practising and have some fun.'

He held up his hands. 'Absolutely.' He leaned forward and caught a whiff of her light perfume. 'How did we get so lucky to meet you?'

She turned her violet gaze towards him and gave him a wink. 'Well, I'm from Scotland, so I guess I must be your lucky white heather.'

His heart gave a swell. It was like the awkwardness had temporarily evacuated the building, and he was here for that. He much preferred it when things were like this.

He still wondered what had caused her reaction before. But since he didn't want to go back there, he wasn't going to ask any questions. If Addy wanted to tell him then she would.

The ward phone rang just as Addy was walking past the nurses' station. 'Cardiology. Charge Nurse Bates.'

'Addy? It's Adhil from Accident and Emergency. We are absolutely slammed. We don't even have a cubicle free. I've triaged a young man in the waiting room who I'm sure has cardiac symptoms. No tests yet. Do you have a consultant free that can see him, if I send him up escorted?'

Addy leaned forward to double check Theo was still on the ward. He was just finishing with a patient in one of the side rooms. 'Yep. Dr Dubois is here. I'll let him know. Give me some details.' She lifted a pen and took some notes. 'Yep, yep…got it. Let the staff know I'll meet them at the elevator.'

She hung up the phone and hurried down the corridor, meeting Theo and Layla as they exited the room. 'We've got an emergency admission coming up, triaged by Adhil in Accident and Emergency, but they don't even have a cubicle to assess him in. Severe chest pain, breathlessness. Twenty-four-year-old male. On his way now. No tests completed as yet.'

She turned to Layla. 'We'll use room three-two-three. Can you bring along the ECG machine and the ultrasound please?'

Theo looked at her. 'Why is Accident and Emergency slammed?'

'RTA, multi-vehicle. Adhil didn't want this young man to get lost in the noise down there when they're already assessing multiple patients.'

Theo nodded. 'Which elevator?'

'South side.'

They both moved quickly and, as soon as the elevator doors opened, they grabbed either side of the trolley.

There was a nurse and porter from Accident and Emergency, and the young man was already on oxygen, with a heart monitor and pulse oximeter in place.

They moved along to the room and transferred him quickly to the bed. The nurse handed over the notes in her hand. 'I'm so sorry, you know we would never usually do this.'

Theo scanned the notes and nodded. 'It's fine, I get it.'

He moved the patient's side. 'Hi, Rio, I'm Dr Dubois, and we're going to take care of you.'

Addy made some quick notes on a chart at the end of the bed. 'BP low, tachycardic and pulse ox ninety.'

From first glance, this was a young, fit-looking man, but it was clear to see he was having trouble breathing and was using all his accessory muscles around the chest to assist.

Theo didn't hesitate—he lifted the transducer from the ultrasound machine that Layla had just wheeled in.

'Rio, I'm going to use this to get a better look at what's going on in your chest. It won't hurt, I'll just slide it across your skin.'

He put some gel on Rio's chest and flicked the machine on.

'How long have you had this chest pain?'

'S-since yesterday,' wheezed Rio.

'What happened yesterday?' asked Theo succinctly.

He was rapidly scanning the structure of the heart and the blood flow through it.

'R-rugby,' wheezed Rio.

Theo's head whipped from the monitor to Rio. 'Did you get hit in the chest?'

Rio nodded.

'Did it hurt straightaway?'

'Took my breath away. But not like this.'

Theo nodded and pointed to the screen. 'Rio, I think you've got something that's called a cardiac tamponade. It can happen for a variety of reasons, but it's likely because you've had a direct injury to the chest. Have you got shorter of breath since the incident?'

Rio nodded again. He looked half-panicked, and half-exhausted.

Theo pointed to another part of the screen. 'There's a sac around your heart called the pericardium. It has two layers and there's normally a little fluid between them. Because you've had an injury to your chest, extra fluid has built up in those layers, meaning that your heart can't pump effectively right now. This is called a pericardial effusion. And what we need to do right now is take the fluid out to reduce the friction on your heart and let it beat properly again.'

Addy had recognised the condition as soon as Theo had put the transducer on Rio's chest. She'd already pulled the emergency trolley into the room, as one of the drawers held the equipment for reducing the pericardial effusion. Cardiac tamponade was often a cardiac emergency and she was sure Theo wouldn't want to delay.

He gave her a nod, and within a few minutes she had the pericardial needle and catheter ready to go as Theo washed his hands and put on some gloves.

Layla kept her eyes on the observations. 'Blood pressure is dropping,' she noted.

Addy drew up the lidocaine, and handed the smaller syringe to Theo, as Layla wiped the area with some antiseptic. 'Just a small prick to numb the area for you,' he said to Rio. 'This might feel a bit tingly on your skin.'

Rio made a face as the lidocaine was injected. Theo waited a few moments until he was sure it had started to take effect.

Addy adjusted some of the cardiac leads to ensure they would have a clear signal while Theo was draining the fluid. Sometimes draining the fluid could lead to a number of extra heartbeats,

or a change in the heart rhythm. It was important
the leads were in the correct position to give them
that information during the procedure.

'Will this hurt?' breathed Rio.

She could see the anxiety on his face and
reached out to hold his hand. 'It might be a little
uncomfortable, but it shouldn't cause you pain.'
She nodded to Theo.

He gave her a hint of a smile. It wasn't obvious.
It was just for her. But it made her heart swell. Because she knew what it meant. He trusted her. He
trusted her as his colleague for this procedure—
to monitor the patient, to keep the situation calm
and to assist in any way she could.

A sense of pride swept over her. And a little
piece of herself slotted into place.

She used to feel like this at her work every
single day. Confident, happy and sure of what
she was doing.

It suddenly struck her how, for a time, that had
been taken from her. When everything had gone
belly up, when Stuart's fraud had made her walls
crumble, and when colleagues had looked at her
with a hint of distrust in their eyes, the one clear
thing that had always been steady in her life had
disintegrated around her.

Coming to Dubai had been part of putting her
life together again. She'd known that. It was why
she'd stepped on the plane.

But she hadn't realised how much his actions—which had absolutely nothing to do with her work—had affected her confidence in her own abilities.

And once she'd got here, it didn't matter what her qualifications were, or what her professional history was. As soon as Dr Gemmill had been annoyed by her challenges, and had her move ward, what little confidence had been left had been stripped from her too.

It was like a lightbulb going off in her head.

She could do this. She had recognised what was wrong with this patient. She knew the procedure well. She knew exactly what would be required, and that the patient needed to be distracted right now, and to hold still during the procedure.

But that one little look from Theo had just made all the pieces fall into place for her.

She sat down next to Rio and started talking to him, taking one of his hands in both of hers, and encouraging him to try and slow his breathing—all while keeping an eye on the monitors.

Theo had a steady pair of hands. Pericardiocentesis needed the steadiest.

Using the ultrasound as a guide, he inserted the needle into the observed gap between the two layers of the pericardial sac. Threading the catheter into place, and then using a three-way tap, he slowly and steadily allowed some of the fluid to drain. It was a delicate process, and everyone in the room knew it.

Addy kept her eyes flicking to the monitor while talking steadily to Rio. His breathing was slowing all the time. It was clear that the gradual reduction in fluid was releasing the pressure on his chest in a positive way.

Layla was keeping her eye on the fluid amount from the other side of the bed. By the time she said the words, 'Three hundred mils...' it was clear Rio was benefiting from the procedure.

He wriggled his shoulders a little and Addy gave his hand a squeeze. 'Try and stay still. This will only take another few minutes, and you'll continue to feel the pressure easing.'

He grimaced but nodded, taking in a long slow breath. The level on his pulse oximeter was gradually rising as the blood started to pump more efficiently around his body and his oxygen levels increased.

Addy took a breath herself. This was one of those procedures where everyone in the room could see the difference the process made. Improvements were rapid for patients.

'A few ectopics,' she said quietly as she kept her eye on the monitor. It was clear Rio had no indication of this. Every person in the world could have ectopic heart beats every day with no ill effects, but in these circumstances it could mean something different.

'Slowing slightly,' said Theo with a nod of his head.

Everyone was watching the monitor. The space between the two layers had reduced, but it was clear there was still some fluid to collect. 'That's been some blow to the chest,' said Theo gently, trying to help distract. 'I'm actually surprised you aren't black and blue.'

Rio pulled a face. 'I never bruise much. I broke a bone once, and apart from the swelling there was no bruising at all. I think, at first, the doctor thought I'd come in with some kind of sprain.' He gave a wide smile. 'He'd been quite dismissive with me, until he saw the X-ray and realised I'd need plates and pins to put my bones back together.'

Theo shot him a smile as he continued with the procedure. 'You must have a good diet, excellent platelets and a good collagen level. All reasons why some people don't bruise as much as others. Genetics can play a part too.'

'So, I should be grateful?'

'Absolutely,' said Theo. 'But, I have to warn you, sometimes if the bruising is deep it takes a few days to develop and show on the surface of the skin.'

Rio took a few more breaths. 'It's definitely starting to feel a bit more comfortable.'

Four hundred and fifty mils, mouthed Layla silently. The amount of fluid was significant.

All eyes went to the monitor where the space between the layers had now reduced. There was always a minimal amount of fluid. It was necessary to remove friction between the two layers as they moved when the heart beat.

Theo watched carefully then turned off the three-way tap. 'Okay Rio. That's us. I'm going to order an X-ray to ensure there's no obvious damage to any of your ribs or lungs after the hit from the rugby ball, and we'll need to monitor you quite closely overnight today and into tomorrow.'

'Why? What can happen?'

'Occasionally fluid can build back up. We might give you some IV fluids to maintain your blood pressure. I'll order some more ECGs throughout the day to ensure everything is going back to normal. I'm also going to order some medicines to keep you comfortable and hopefully stop any inflammation of the heart.'

'But I can play rugby again, can't I?'

Theo caught Addy's smile as she shook her head and gave a short laugh.

'Can I do this one?' she asked.

Theo nodded as he snapped off his gloves and moved to the sink to wash his hands.

Addy looked at Rio. 'You can absolutely play rugby again, but only when Dr Dubois says it's safe. We need to make sure your heart has completely recovered before you start vigorous exercise again. Given your age and fitness level it will likely only be a few weeks.'

'So, I'm benched for the next two weeks?' He'd jumped on the word 'few'.

She wagged her finger at him. 'Remember, we still have to check you have no other injuries to your ribs, or your lungs. That could also affect your recovery time.' She raised her eyebrows at him. 'It could be up to a month.'

He groaned and leaned his head back on his pillow, as if this were the worst thing in the world. It was clear Rio didn't realise just how serious a cardiac tamponade could be.

'Your heart is the most important muscle in your body. It's just been under a lot of stress. You need to let it recover. You only get one,' she added with a wink. 'Remember how sick you felt less than half an hour ago.'

'Okay,' he groaned, but it was good-natured. He looked back at Addy. 'You seem like you'll be fit enough to tell my coach that.' He gave an approving nod. 'The Scottish accent will probably keep him in his place.'

Addy held out her hand. 'Give me his number. He'll be putty in my hands.'

She felt good as she phoned the coach and told him about Rio's injury and recovery time. She understood exactly why Rio had wanted her to phone, because of the coach's initial reaction and the fact he thought he could 'negotiate' Rio's recovery. But Addy had dealt with people like this before. She made sure that he knew he would have to be patient and wait for Rio to get the all-clear. She only had to mention the words 'insurance' and 'liability' for him to pay attention.

After that, she spoke to some other relatives whose family matriarch had suffered from a severe MI and required coronary artery bypass. They were so grateful for the care and attention their family member had received, and Addy was touched by their sincerity and admiration.

By the time Rio's chest X-ray was reported on, and his first set of ECGs had been repeated, both of them were over their shift time. Rio's blood pressure had stabilised now he was on some IV fluids, and his immediate pain had eased. He was eating some toast by the time they were ready to leave.

Max chatted easily when collected from daycare, and Theo invited Addy to join them for dinner. They debated the contents of his fridge, before she returned to her own apartment and brought back some chicken to make some pasta for them all.

He came and stood behind her, sliding his arms around her waist as she was stirring the pasta and sauce in a pot. She leaned back against him. 'I feel as if I need to make a disclaimer about my cooking skills not always being the best.'

'And you think mine are?'

The warmth of his body permeated her thin T-shirt. She liked it. It felt natural. It felt right. 'I can promise faithfully that the chicken is properly cooked. But after that? It's just a chance we all have to take.'

'Maybe long-term we should try and teach Max to cook. It could save us all.'

A little tremor went through her skin. Long-term. He'd said the words 'long-term', and that was clearly how he was starting to think now.

It delighted her. It excited her. And it also terrified her.

Was this too soon? Because part of her head said yes, but her heart had a mind of its own.

She liked the routine they were falling into. She liked being able to look across the ward and communicate with Theo without actually saying anything.

She waited until the pasta had been served and eaten, and Max was in bed, before she finally took a breath to speak.

She was lying against him on the sofa, drinking a glass of wine, and staring out at the beautiful night sky. 'Today's the best day I've had in a long time,' she admitted. It was time to open up—even just a little.

She sensed his body reacting a little. 'What do you mean?'

His arm was around her neck, and his hand draped down towards her chest. She started tracing her fingers along the back of his hand. 'I mean today, on the ward, at work, was the happiest I've been in a long time.'

'You mean since you got here? Do you think you've settled in?'

She paused and licked her lips, wondering how much to say. 'Yes and no. I've never done anything wrong at work. But my confidence was knocked at the last place. I'd always been super proud of my job, and what I did, but then some things happened, and I started to hate going to work. To hate the place I'd always loved.'

He shifted as he tried to get a better position to look at her. 'Did something happen at work?'

She shook her head. 'No, that's the sad thing. Some stuff happened outside of work. It wasn't anything to do with work at all. But I felt as if people looked at me differently, treated me differently. And the place I'd loved working at, and been confident in, made me feel as if I were under a microscope. I second-guessed myself when I'd always been happy with my decisions and clinical care.'

'Couldn't you speak to someone? Didn't you have a boss you could go to?'

She sighed. 'It just didn't work like that. The old consultant I worked with—he never listened to anything outside work. So I know he had no issues with me. But you know what a hospital is like. Rumours come from outside, and then everyone's looking at you. People stop talking when you come near—and you know you've been the topic of conversation.'

'But…' she could tell he was speaking carefully '…if this is all external, and nothing to do with work, people had no business making you feel uncomfortable. You should have spoken to HR, asked them to stop the rumours.'

She'd only given him a tiny hint of what she'd been through. But he was taking it so well, being supportive and not judgemental at all. A tiny voice in her head urged her to say more—to tell him all about the debt, the fraud and the current issues with the police.

But it was too much to tell him all that. After a tense week, they were just back to where they wanted to be. She'd asked him to be patient, and he'd agreed. The last thing she wanted to do now was spoil the moment they were in.

So she gave a soft laugh and laid her head back against his shoulder. 'You know it doesn't work like that. It's all "he said, she said" and you can't really prove anything. There's just tension—an atmosphere—and the place that always felt like home feels different.'

He ran a finger down her cheek. 'So, how do you feel about being here?'

She bit her bottom lip and looked into his brown eyes. 'Better. Now I feel better.' She pulled a face. 'For a while, it was touch and go.'

'You mean with Dr Gemmill?'

She gave a nod. 'It was like jumping out of the frying pan and into the fire. I'm too passionate about patient care not to say anything. When they moved my ward, I thought they were actually going to sack me.'

Now he did sit up straight. 'Honestly?'

She nodded. 'And I didn't really know anyone. I didn't know who to speak to. I'd just got here. I didn't have any friends.'

'You could have spoken to me.'

She gave him a sad smile. 'But I thought you were on his side. I thought you agreed with him.'

He sighed and pulled her closer. 'I'm sorry you thought that. I was trying to offer advice. I didn't appreciate that you might be feeling like that.'

He stroked the side of her face. 'They gave you the job because they know you're capable and competent. Your references must have been good—so it's clear they thought you could do the job. Do you know they interviewed twenty candidates for your role?'

'What?' Now it was her turn to sit up. She was totally shocked.

He smiled. 'Spira is a competitive place. People want to work here. But they want the best.'

She sat back again. 'Wow, I didn't know that.'

He pulled her closer to him. 'And it's not just Spira that wants you. Max and I want you too.'

She shivered. A good shiver. One of excitement and anticipation.

'You do?'

He nodded. 'I know things have been a bit tense between us up until now. I guess I didn't know how you were feeling, and I guess you also realise how I'm hanging in here by the seat of my pants when it comes to Max.'

'He's a great kid, Theo,' she said. She couldn't hide the affection in her voice. 'I love being around him.'

'And he loves being around you. He talks about you all the time.'

'He does?' She pressed her lips together. 'This last week I missed being around him. It's why I went to see him at daycare.'

'I figured,' he said gently. 'So, where does that leave us?'

She smiled. 'Where do you want it to leave us?'

His deep brown eyes looked at her carefully. 'I want us to be around each other. I want you in both of our lives, but I don't want to rush you into anything if you're not ready.'

She reached over and put her hand on his chest. 'I didn't expect this. I didn't come here expecting to find someone. Or two someones. But this is what I want,' she said, her stomach slightly knotted. 'I want us to be together too.'

He bent forward and kissed her lips lightly. 'What about Max? You know how I feel about things.'

She closed her eyes and smiled as his lips danced across her cheek. 'I love him,' she said easily. 'In an ideal world we would have dated longer before I met Max. But I get that you come together.' She gave a shrug. 'I never had a plan around children. I never thought no. I just figured children would happen at the right time in my life.' Her eyes opened and fixed on his. 'I guess the world just knows better than we do.'

He ran his fingers through her hair. 'So, you're happy. We can take some time and figure out things together. We'll have to be up front and tell HR that we're dating before someone else does.'

'I'm happy to do that.' She laughed. 'What's the worst that can happen—they'll move me again?'

His brow furrowed. 'You don't honestly think they'd do that?'

'I don't know what the rules are. Some hospitals don't like staff dating and working together. Just in case something goes wrong and they cover for each other.'

'But that's not going to happen. I'd prefer to be up front with people. If they want to give us a set of rules for the workplace, then that's fine.'

She licked her lips. 'So, what about Max? What do we tell Max?'

He paused for a moment. She could imagine the number of conflicting thoughts that were going through his brain.

She put her hand on Theo's chest. 'How about we don't do anything at all? We see each other. We spend time in each other's apartments.' She raised her eyebrows. 'You might even let me have a sleepover. But we don't sit him down and make a big thing of it. We let it develop naturally. He's used to us being around each other. We let *him* get used to us.'

Theo gave a few small nods, and Addy continued. 'And if you notice anything—if he's having nightmares again, or his behaviour changes—we can take a few steps back.'

His shoulders relaxed a little and she knew that he must have been worried.

'Let's take this easy,' he said. 'Easy on us, easy

on Max. If I'm too intense, if I'm not intense enough—just tell me. If I don't sleep, I know that I get short-tempered.'

'Is this our cue to tell each other all our faults?'

He grinned. 'Go on then.'

'I sometimes snore. So, I might be responsible for you not getting enough sleep.'

He leaned over and whispered in her ear. 'That better not be the only way you keep me up all night.'

She snaked her arms around his neck. 'That's something we could discuss together.'

There was a gleam in his eyes. 'When would you like to start?'

She pulled him on top of her as she slid down the sofa. 'How about now?'

CHAPTER ELEVEN

THE WARD WAS almost full. Only two beds were free, and both were assigned to patients coming in for investigations or procedures.

The last few weeks had been perfect. They'd seen each other every day and night. Max appeared entirely comfortable. He loved snuggling up on the sofa with Addy and telling her his daycare stories. They'd visited an aquarium, a water park and a mall with a special area for kids.

Things were so easy between them. Theo had learned her favourite foods and movies, and she'd learned his. They laughed together, supported each other and encouraged Max's learning in any way they could.

For the first time since he'd got Max, Theo didn't feel on his own. It felt instead like he was building a relationship and a family, and that made him proud and happy at the same time.

Occasionally his head flipped back to what little that she'd told him about her old job and loss of confidence. She never mentioned past relationships, or what had caused those tensions at the hospital. But she'd asked him to be patient with her. So he had to believe, if there was anything important, she would tell him when she was ready—even if he had to wait a bit longer.

His pager sounded, and he answered immediately. It was his secretary. 'Dr Dubois,' she said, 'you asked me to update you on Isabel Aurelis. I spoke to her yesterday after all her assigned tests were completed. She was supposed to report today for admission, but she's over an hour late. I've tried her mobile with no response.'

Theo felt an uncomfortable prickle go up his spine. 'Where does she stay?'

His secretary read off the address.

'And do we have a next of kin for Isabel, a parent or friend?'

'Yes, I have contact details for both of her parents.'

'Can you try them please?'

He replaced the received and walked down the corridor to find Addy. She was chatting with one of the other cardiology consultants over preparing a patient for a procedure.

Theo rested his hands on his hips. 'One of Dr Gemmill's patients was supposed to come in today. She hasn't appeared.'

The other consultant gave a soft laugh. 'They've

probably gone to the tennis club or the cricket club instead.'

Theo shook his head. 'Unlikely. She's only twenty-one. Previous admission for investigations of Wolff-Parkinson-White.'

The other consultant's eyebrows raised. 'The one who arrested and caused the ruckus?'

Theo nodded and Addy answered. 'Well, we all know it was me that caused the ruckus, because she was admitted with no real details. But that's a worry. Is there any chance she's taken unwell?'

He sighed. 'My secretary is trying to get hold of her next of kin. I'm hoping she's a young lady with a better offer who forgot about her admission today.'

'Has she had any other episodes?' the other consultant asked.

'That's the problem,' said Theo. 'She's had a number, but was still under Dr Gemmill. I had to contact her to try and get her tests all completed since her symptoms were worsening.'

His pager sounded—he walked to the wall and picked up the phone. 'Yes, okay, I see. Where are they? No one? Okay. How would they feel about us visiting?' He met Addy's violet gaze. She knew exactly how worried he was.

He hung up the phone. 'Her parents are in Gibraltar. They've tried her too, and one of her friends couldn't get hold of her this morning.'

'Are you going to send someone to her address?' asked the other consultant, his face grave.

'Actually...' said Theo, looking at him.

'Go.' He gave a wave of his hand. 'I can cover here. Who will you take with you?'

'Me,' said Addy. 'I'll give the keycards for the medicine trolley to Layla, and let the sister in the next ward know where we're going.'

She ran to the office and grabbed a few things, sticking them in a bag, before joining Theo at the elevator a few minutes later. They grabbed one of the porters to borrow a Spira staff car; and he drove them the short distance across the city.

Isabel stayed in a complex much more luxurious than the one the hospital hosted them in. A concierge was waiting at the door for them.

'You are the doctors from Spira?'

Theo nodded and the man strode swiftly towards another elevator. 'This takes us straight to the penthouse,' he said. 'I was just about to go up. Mr and Mrs Aurelis have phoned.'

The elevator was speedier than normal and Theo realised on the ascent that there were no other buttons. This must be exclusively for the penthouse.

There was an outer door that the concierge opened with his sensor. 'Ms Aurelis?' he shouted in a booming voice that took both Theo and Addy by surprise.

He started walking through the hall to the main living room, which was empty. It had vast views and exquisite furniture. 'There are four bedrooms, a study, three bathrooms, a dining room, kitchen, dressing room and laundry room,' he said briskly, waving his hand. Theo and Addy took that as their cue to help with the search.

They both ducked into other rooms. Theo was first into a bedroom, walking right round the whole room and checking inside the adjoining bathroom. Next was a study—he even checked under the desk.

Then he heard a shout. 'In here!'

It was Addy, and by the time he'd raced through she was on the floor of another bathroom. Isabel had clearly been about to either shower or bathe, as a number of glass bottles had broken and spilled liquid on the floor. Addy had covered her with a bathrobe and a towel while she checked her airway, breathing and circulation.

'She's breathing...it's shallow, but it's there. Her heart rate is very fast.' Addy reached into her bag and pulled out the portable monitor that she'd brought with her, fastening a few electrodes to Isabel's chest.

Theo was down on his knees next to her. He gave Isabel a little shake on the shoulder.

'Isabel, can you hear us? It's Dr Dubois and

Charge Nurse Bates from Spira Hospital. You've had a turn, and we've come to check on you.'

His eyes flicked to the monitor now the rhythm was showing on the screen. 'Rate two-twenty, SVT, we have no way of knowing how long she's been like this.'

He looked back across to Addy, since Isabel hadn't responded yet. 'Do you have a BP cuff?'

She nodded. 'It's manual,' she said apologetically, pulling a stethoscope and BP cuff from the bag.

He fastened it around Isabel's upper arm, inflated the cuff and listened with the stethoscope at her inner elbow. 'Eighty over fifty. Not great.' He pulled some adenosine from his pocket and looked over his shoulder at their porter, who was standing at the door. 'Get us an ambulance please. We're taking this patient in with us directly.'

He injected the adenosine, hoping to reduce Isabel's heart rate and stabilise things. As he looked up, he realised the concierge looked stricken. 'Can you call Isabel's parents back? Let them know we've got her and we're taking her back to Spira for a possible procedure this afternoon? They can call us later for more information.'

Addy had her head low, whispering in Isabel's ear as they continued to monitor her. 'Cardiac ablation?' she said.

'Unless we see a direct improvement,' he said.

'We can't leave her like this. And it has a good success rate.'

They waited patiently. Isabel became a little more aware of her surroundings but was still semi-conscious. Her heart rate slowed only a little, and it became clear they were going to have to continue her treatment.

By the time the ambulance arrived, they were ready to leave straightaway. Addy had grabbed some things from Isabel's cupboards and bathroom, equipping her stay for a few nights. The concierge locked up the penthouse and said he'd arrange a cleaning service.

Addy had phoned through to Spira to set up the cath lab for an emergency ablation procedure.

They went straight through Accident and Emergency to the cath lab. There were few staff available to prepare Isabel, so Addy completed the normal admission paperwork with all her details and medical history, and drew an emergency set of bloods.

By the time she'd finished, Theo was ready to start the procedure. Addy threw on a set of scrubs, standing in the background to observe.

It was clear Theo had done this many times. He inserted a sheath into a vessel near Isabel's groin before threading the catheter up towards her heart. The catheter electrodes—long thin wires moved up into the heart—were then delicately put into place as they all watched the whole process via a camera. It was a delicate procedure, because Theo had to find the abnormal tissue that was sending the rogue electrical impulses, then make sure the electrode catheter was in exactly the right spot before sending an energy pulse that destroyed the rogue tissue. As they watched the monitor, they could tell the procedure had been a success—Isabel's heart rate dropped and reverted to a normal rhythm.

Addy smiled as she heard the collective sigh of relief from everyone in the room. She moved over next to the trolley. 'I'll take her through to recovery,' she volunteered with a nod to the anaesthetist.

Isabel quickly started to come round. She was still monitored and on oxygen for a period of time, but her blood pressure improved and her heart rate stayed in a regular rhythm, at a normal rate.

An hour later, Addy took her up to the ward.

The consultant who'd been left on shift smiled but raised his eyebrows at her, handing her a pile of sticky notes. 'Mr and Mrs Aurelis are very anxious to speak to one of you. They're flying back from Gibraltar but wanted to speak to someone before their flight took off.'

Addy smiled and put the notes in her pocket.

'I'll phone them as soon as I have Isabel settled in her room.'

Layla joined her, and Addy gave her a handover, arranging for Isabel to get some food. 'She'll be staying for overnight monitoring and will be reviewed in the morning, with a view to potential discharge, all being well.'

Addy tapped her pocket. 'Isabel, I'm going to phone your mum and dad. Layla, warn the night shift that Isabel might have some late-night visitors.'

She shot them both a smile, then spent the next thirty minutes on the phone to some anxious but very grateful patients.

Theo appeared, to write up his notes, and heard the tail end of the conversation. He grinned when she finished. 'Well, this has been a bit of an unusual day.'

'It has been.' She nodded in agreement and then looked at the clock. 'Do you want me to pick up something for dinner, or collect Max from daycare?'

His eyes darted to the clock and he groaned. 'Pick up Max, please, and I'll sort out dinner. Do you want my key card?'

She shook her head. 'I'll take him to mine. You can give us a knock when you finish up.'

'Thank you.' He smiled at her, and her heart gave a little leap. The crinkles around his brown eyes and the expression on his face touched every part of her. It was the casualness. The sureness of each other. That fire still burning between them. And the trust.

No matter how they'd got here, she was absolutely sure about what she wanted for her future. It had two names. Theo and Max.

She still hadn't told him everything. The calls between her and her lawyer had increased as events continued to get worse back home. She definitely didn't want to leave Dubai, but it was now becoming a distinct possibility. Anxiety pricked at her that she hadn't told Theo everything, but she knew she would...as soon as she had a clear plan for what would happen next. The last thing she wanted to do was put any extra worry on him.

She was learning how to be a mum by default and was absolutely loving it. She'd asked some friends at the book group she was attending for a few hints on things, and they'd been more than delighted to help. From making food a bit more child friendly, to helping their attention span, to dealing with tantrums, and getting them to help around the house safely. Some of their suggestions were things she hadn't even considered, and she'd enjoyed feeding back to them too. Making new friends as an adult was always slightly awkward, particularly when she'd no starting point in

Dubai, but the book group was an absolute god-send. Who'd known reading romance, crime and historical novels could teach so much?

Addy swung her bag over her shoulder, had a quick check to make sure no one was looking in the office, then gave Theo a kiss on the cheek. She gave him a wave as she headed to daycare.

Max was sitting scrunched up in a corner. Usually he was full of beans and waiting for one of them to appear.

'Okay, honey?' she asked.

He nodded but kept his head down.

She checked with a member of staff. 'Everything okay with Max?'

The staff member nodded. 'He's been a bit quiet this afternoon, but he says nothing is wrong.'

Addy thanked her and collected his backpack. 'Come on. We'll go home to mine until Dad finishes work.'

That was another thing that had changed in the last few weeks. Max had started to call Theo 'Dad' instead of Theo. Neither of them had tried to correct him, and she could see how secretly proud he was of the title.

They walked home, rather slowly, but the few times she offered to carry Max he refused.

When they reached her apartment, she dumped their stuff and settled him on the sofa. 'Let me check your temperature,' she said quickly, feeling his forehead. He didn't feel warm…

As she checked his temperature, she noticed her answering machine blinking red.

Max temperature was fine. But he was rubbing his eyes. 'I'm sleepy.'

'Okay, honey,' she said, picking up a nearby blanket. 'Did you do a lot in daycare today?'

He gave a scowl. 'Not really. Just fought with Rueben. I don't like him.'

Addy knelt down in front of him, watching as he lay his head on a cushion. If something significant happened, the daycare staff would always tell them. 'What did you fight about?' she asked carefully.

'A dinosaur.'

Addy waited for more information, but none came. 'Doesn't daycare teach you to share, or take turns?'

Max kept scowling. 'I'd only just got it. I told him he could have it later.'

'And what did he do?' asked Addy, hoping she got a good answer.

'He pushed me.'

'He did?'

Max nodded. 'So I bit him.'

Addy felt her stomach flip over. 'Oh, no, Max. We don't bite other people. That's naughty.'

If daycare had missed this altercation, there

was a chance Rueben might go home with a bite mark somewhere, and that would likely create havoc. She should really phone them.

Max pulled his blanket up. 'I'm tired,' he said again, and closed his eyes.

Addy's mouth was half open, and she was ready to say something, but she took a deep breath and closed it, touching his little head once again.

She would have to tell Theo when he got back. Max had generally been well-behaved around her. She'd only seen him throw a temper tantrum once, and she knew he'd been overtired at that point.

But biting was serious, and her stomach churned as she thought how she would feel if Max had shown her a bite mark on his skin today.

She stood up and stretched. There was no point tackling this now. She'd talk it through with Theo once he got home. If Max had a sleep right now, he might be in a better mood once he woke up.

She moved over to the phone and remembered there was a message. She pressed the button to listen. It was Laura, her lawyer. 'Hi, Addy. Listen, I'm sorry, but things have taken a bit of a turn. Can you phone me urgently please?'

Addy's stomach lurched. She felt a wave of panic.

She pressed the buttons to dial Laura, her

hands shaking so much that she put the phone on speaker mode rather than holding it.

'It's Addy.'

'We have a problem.'

'What do you mean?'

'The new inspector is threatening to put a warrant out for your arrest.'

'What?' Her legs wobbled and she started to shake. 'How on earth can he do that?'

'He claims you've been uncooperative about being interviewed.'

'I've sent him my shifts three times. He's never asked me to meet him.'

'I went through that with him, but he says you're being deliberately uncooperative.'

'Surely it's his job to arrange a time that suits? This job at Spira is different from other posts I've had. In theory I have to be available seven days a week, twenty-four hours a day. But the reality is I have to be there for the busy periods. And since most of Spira's cardiac admissions are arranged, that's usually Monday to Friday between eight and five. So that makes me unavailable for the inspector during those hours.'

'I know that,' said Laura. 'But it seems that he's talked to Stuart again and dreamed up some more charges.'

'Like what?' She could feel cold sweat breaking out on her skin.

'Fraud, extortion, cyber-crime, theft and corruption.'

'What?' Her throat was dry and her brain was going into panic mode.

'How can this be happening? I've offered to speak to him. He's conjuring up charges without having a clear picture of what went on.'

'Addy?'

The voice cut through the noise in her brain. Theo was standing in the doorway with a look of confusion on his face.

For a moment, all words left her mind—it almost seemed as if she'd lost the ability to talk.

Laura kept talking. 'He's serious, Addy. He wants to put out a warrant for your arrest. He might even contact your employers. I'm thinking you'll have to come back to Scotland.'

Addy turned away from the phone to see Theo's face.

'I… I can explain,' she stuttered.

'Where's Max?' he asked, his face blank.

'He's sleeping,' she said, pointing to the sofa that she'd turned to face the window.

'Sleeping? Why is he sleeping?' Theo crossed the space in a few strides.

'He said he was tired. And daycare said he'd been quiet this afternoon. We talked when we got home and he told me he'd been fighting and bit another kid.'

She kept on glancing at the phone, conscious that Laura would hear her. This wasn't how she wanted to deal with things.

'What?' Theo's face whipped around to look at her again as he knelt at the sofa. 'You should have phoned me.'

'I would have, but…' Her voice tailed off.

Yes, she probably should have phoned him, but she hadn't wanted to make a big deal out of it in front of Max, and had hoped they would've had a chance to talk privately.

'Max?' Theo's voice was quiet as he tried to shake Max awake.

Addy started to speak. 'Laura, this isn't a good time right now. I'll need to call you—'

'Max!' Theo's voice was sharp now, and it stopped her mid-sentence. 'Max!'

She recognised the tone and ran over to his side. He was shaking Max sharply now, but Max was definitely not waking up.

'What's wrong with him? What have you done to him?'

'What? Nothing. He was talking to me earlier. I checked his temperature…it was fine.' She put her hand onto the little body and tried to rouse him too.

Theo started running his hands over Max's body. Touching his stomach, his limbs, then pulling up his eyelids to check his pupils.

Max gave the tiniest groan, but that was it.

There was no question. Max was unconscious.

Theo ran his hands around his son's head and stopped short, his head snapping around to her. 'What's this lump?'

'What lump?' She tried to get a look, but Theo was blocking her way.

His voice was like steel. 'My son has a lump on his head and he's unconscious. What have you done?'

Fear gripped her, along with a wave of anger. 'I told you! He was fighting with another kid at daycare. But he never said he hit his head. He didn't complain about his head at all. He just said he was tired. Daycare didn't say anything at all.'

Her brain was whirling. She reached over to touch Max's head, instantly terrified when she touched the lump. It was definite. But his skin was unbroken, there was no blood.

'What do we do?' she asked, all her nursing background flooding out the window, leaving her scared and panicked.

'*We* do nothing,' Theo spat out as he gathered his son in his arms. Then he clearly had second thoughts. 'Phone an ambulance. I'll meet them at the front door.'

Her trembling fingers cut the call to Laura without a word and dialled for an ambulance. She gave the details, telling them Max was unconscious and his father would meet them at the door.

All of a sudden she was furious that she hadn't taken Theo's key earlier. If they'd been in his apartment she could have gathered some things for them to take to the hospital. She grabbed Max's backpack from earlier, her own jacket and bag, and ran to the elevator. She had to know. She had to know that Max was going to be okay.

But by the time she reached the ground floor, the ambulance was already there, and Max and Theo were bundled inside, Theo talking to the paramedic. As she scrambled to get closer Theo saw her and his eyes cut her dead.

'Stay,' was the only word he said before the back doors of the ambulance were slammed.

The siren sounded. Her legs buckled and sent her onto the pavement as the two people she loved most in the world disappeared, leaving her with no idea of their future.

CHAPTER TWELVE

THEO DID HIS absolute best not to vomit all over the back of the ambulance or get in the way of the paramedic who was tending to his son.

The overwhelming urge to panic and rant and rave was right on the tip of his tongue. He'd heard a colleague say once that when someone had crashed into her car, with her children in the back, she'd panicked, checked her children were okay and grabbed them and ran—not even talking to the person who had crashed into her. The calmest doctor he'd ever known had told him that, in that moment, she couldn't talk to anyone, and just ran to a friend's house that was nearby.

Theo had been bewildered by her words. Now he understood them entirely.

They arrived at Spira within minutes. A few of the staff recognised him and one of the Accident and Emergency doctors came over straight away.

'Theo? What's wrong?'

'This is my son, Max, he's three. He's unconscious and has a lump at the back of his head.' He struggled with the next words as a wash of guilt embraced him. 'My…friend picked him up from daycare. He was fine but quiet. Daycare didn't report anything, but my friend said that Max told her he'd been in a fight today. He was tired. She let him sleep.'

'How long has he been sleeping?'

Theo took in a deep breath, thinking what time Addy had picked him up. 'It will be about two hours, maybe longer.'

He should have picked Max up. Would he have noticed there was something wrong?

'Any vomiting? Irritability?'

'I don't think so…'

He said this just as Max, who was on his side, vomited everywhere.

'Let me do some neuro obs and take a good look at him,' said the doctor, wheeling the trolley into the resus room.

The staff moved quickly, almost without saying a word to each other. They knew exactly what they were doing. They took his observations, filling out a neuro chart and shining a light into Max's pupils. Then they took some time to examine the bump at the back of Max's head.

'I really need more information about what happened at daycare today,' said the doctor.

'So do I,' muttered Theo.

'And I'm sorry, but I have to ask the question.

Is there any chance he could have been injured by your friend?'

Theo had put a hand on the wall behind him. After everything he'd just heard on that call, all the secrets Addy had been keeping from him, did he think she could have hurt Max? Why had she been keeping secrets? Why on earth were the police pursuing her, and why did they think she was guilty of fraud? He had so many questions tumbling around in his brain. He'd thought it was wrong to push her. He'd promised to be patient. Now it seemed there was so much he didn't know. But did any of that mean she would hurt Max?

'No,' he said. 'It's Addison Bates, the charge nurse from my ward. She would never hurt Max.'

The doctor disappeared for a few moments and came back. 'He's still unconscious. I'm taking him for an emergency scan.'

Theo knew he should try to get more information from the daycare, but there was no way he was leaving his son's side. He strode along next to the trolley as they wheeled it through for the scan, and sat outside as the detailed scan took place.

He knew, in these circumstances, they would report on it immediately.

Fifteen minutes later, the doctor joined him outside the waiting room. 'Dr Baz, the neurosurgeon, is on his way to Theatre. Max has an acute subdural haemorrhage. They need to release the pressure.'

Theo was thankful he was sitting down—his whole body crumpled and he put his head in his hands.

'Is there someone I can call for you?' asked the other doctor.

After a few minutes, Theo took a deep breath and sat up straight. 'No,' he said with conviction. 'No one at all.'

Addy was pacing. He'd told her to stay. He didn't want her there. He'd asked her what she'd done to Max—he'd actually said those words out loud, and now her heart was broken. She had no idea how much he'd heard of her call to Laura. She had to presume he'd heard everything. But there had been no chance to discuss it. No chance to tell him about her evil ex and his actions, that she'd done nothing wrong—at any point.

But she had. She had done something wrong. She hadn't taken the opportunity to tell Theo what had happened in her past. He'd told her his past, and how he'd got Max. He'd shared with her openly, and she hadn't paid him the same courtesy. All to save face? All because she was scared she'd look foolish?

She wanted to turn back the clock so badly right now. But not for her. For Max. Why hadn't she paid better attention? Why hadn't she at least phoned the daycare to ask what had happened?

Max was her favourite little person on the planet, and she'd failed him.

She had to know. She had to know how he was. She knew that by calling she might put fellow colleagues in a difficult position. Some knew that she and Theo were together.

She picked up the phone. 'It's Addy,' she said when someone she knew answered. 'How's Max?'

The person paused a little. 'He's just gone to Theatre. Are you coming in?'

She held back the retch in her throat. 'What kind of injury is it?'

'Subdural,' came the reply. 'Theo looks terrible. Where are you?'

Where was she? On the floor of her apartment, with her head between her knees.

'On my way,' she said.

No matter what the consequences, she had to be there. She had to be there for her boys.

CHAPTER THIRTEEN

Two days passed in a blur. Max's surgery was successful. He was fitted with a shunt for twenty-four hours, and it was removed when the surgeon was sure the swelling and bleeding had passed.

Theo never left his bedside. Someone from the daycare came down to see him, distraught after they'd viewed security tapes that had shown the two three-year-olds clearly fighting, and the other boy pushing Max over so the back of his head struck the corner of a table. He jumped up and bit the boy in retaliation, and then the two boys started playing together again. It had all been over in seconds, and none of the staff had noticed at the time.

At first Theo was confused. Of course, he would have gone to them at a later date and asked for an explanation, but the manager gently explained that Addy had gone to see them. She'd let them know about Max, and asked them to supply Theo with more details in case the surgeon asked.

He was stunned. She'd asked to get in a few

times and he'd just said no. He couldn't think about her, or anything that he'd heard in that call, because his primary focus had to be Max.

When Max opened his eyes and smiled at him, it felt as if the elephant on his shoulders had finally left. For the first time in two days he could breathe. And then he cried. Max had rapidly become his whole world. He hadn't asked for this. He wasn't even sure he wanted it at first. But welcoming Max into his life had been the best thing he'd ever done. Now he understood why people who were parents would do anything for their kids. It didn't matter that he wasn't Max's biological dad. He felt it, inside, and he knew that would never change.

So when Max finally started speaking and asked, 'Where's Addy?' the pain in Theo's heart was so acute he felt he couldn't speak.

Max loved Addy. And so did Theo.

But he'd been so blindsided by things these last few days he hadn't been able to think straight.

He cringed as he remembered some of the things he'd said to her—what he might even have accused her of. It didn't matter that he'd done it without thinking, it was an unforgivable thing to do. He understood that now.

He stroked the top of Max's head. 'Don't worry, honey. I'll find her later and bring her here.'

When Max fell asleep again, he ducked out

to head to the apartments. He tried her door but got no answer. He tried her phone too, but it went straight to message. He hesitated for a few moments, wondering what on earth to say, before finally hanging up and deciding to try again later.

As he went back downstairs, he approached the concierge, who immediately asked how Max was. Theo filled him in and then asked the question. 'Have you seen Addy?'

The concierge looked uncomfortable. 'She's gone—she didn't tell you?'

'What?' Theo felt as if the floor had just opened beneath him.

The concierge nodded. 'She went to the airport. Said she had to go back to the UK to sort some things out.'

'But she's coming back?' He could hear the edge in his tone.

'I'm sorry, Dr Dubois, I don't know. The apartment is still in her name, but she didn't tell me her intentions.'

Theo gave a nod and went back upstairs. He looked in despair at her closed door before opening his own. He walked over to the floor-to-ceiling windows.

A world of possibilities was out there, but he didn't want them without Addy. They were a family. They were meant to be together. He should never have snapped at her. He should have let her visit Max. Now he didn't know if he would get that chance.

His heart felt as if it had been ripped in two. How on earth could he explain to Max that she'd gone?

A tear slid down his face as he turned away from the window. He'd made the biggest mistake of his life, and he had no idea how to fix it.

CHAPTER FOURTEEN

BY THE TIME she landed at Glasgow the rage had built inside her for hours. Laura had strongly advised her to come home. She'd booked them an interview with the new inspector. Addy had left Dubai knowing that Max was out of danger, but she hadn't been able to see him. She longed to see his face again, and longed for a chance to talk to Theo.

But first she had to deal with the chaos that Stuart King had caused in her life again. And she was done with it. Laura kept trying to talk her down, but Addy had taken as much as she could. 'I've travelled nearly five thousand miles to sort this out. You can bet I'll answer the inspector's questions, and then let him know I have no intention of letting this man ruin my life again. My patience is done. I've left behind a three-year-old that I love who's recovering from brain surgery to be here. If this man is so gullible that he believes what a liar and fraudster says—just because he has the gift of the gab—then he's clearly a fool.'

'Please don't say that,' pleaded Laura.

'I might,' bit back Addy. 'You're just here to advise.'

She spent two days being questioned. Things were heated. But Addy could answer every question, explain every transaction. Give proof of shifts and of being in other places when, apparently, she'd applied for loans or remortgaged her house. She was angry. But she was also precise and consistent.

By the time she left, she had been guaranteed, in-person, that there would no investigation into her, no charges and no further need to remain in the country. But that wasn't enough for Addy. 'What about Stuart King? This man has tried to ruin my life twice. He can't be allowed to do this to anyone else—even though the likelihood is that he already has.'

The inspector assured her that they now had multiple pieces of evidence that would allow them to bring charges against Stuart King. He would be arrested in the next few days.

The relief was immense, but so was the sadness.

Theo might never speak to her again. She might never get to be in Max's life. She'd been hurt beyond belief when Theo had uttered the words *'What have you done?'* But she also understood he was panicking, and he'd walked into a situation that she'd had time and opportunity to tell him about, but she'd chosen not to.

He had a right to be angry, he had a right to be suspicious. But how could she continue at Spira if he was going to hate the ground she walked on?

It would be unbearable, because she loved him—she loved them both. They were her perfect family. And life would never be the same if she didn't have them alongside her.

So, she pulled out the last of her recent savings and bought a ticket back to Dubai. Worst-case scenario, she could pick up the rest of her things and give formal notice to HR.

Best-case scenario? She couldn't even dare to hope…

CHAPTER FIFTEEN

IT HAD BEEN five long days. He'd watched her
apartment every day and asked the concierge
if he'd heard anything. He'd also promised the
concierge that the item he'd had delivered to her
apartment was entirely expected. She'd just forgotten to let the concierge know.

His senses were on high alert, and his door
had been ajar the whole time. So, when he finally
heard some footsteps in the corridor, his heart
missed a few beats.

Max was home now, and sleeping peacefully.
He'd made a full recovery, but Theo was off sick
for the rest of this week, to give Max some recu-
peration time and allow him to get fully back to
normal. He'd swithered about leaving altogether
and not using the Spira daycare again, but he
was satisfied by the explanation from the staff,
and their promises. Max had even asked when he
could play with this Rueben again.

His breath caught in his throat as he heard the
steps. They didn't slow at all as they passed his

doorway. He only made it to the corridor in time to see her door open and hear the gasp of shock.

He moved swiftly. Her hands were still at her mouth as she took in the giant patchwork sofa in place of the previous standard cream one.

He spoke in the quietest voice possible. 'Thought it might hide the baked bean stains if Max and I come here.'

She spun around to look at him. He could see everything in her eyes. She looked weary—exhausted, even. Then she swayed a little and he caught her elbows.

'Addison?'

She shook her head and took a few deep breaths. When she lifted her head again there were tears in her eyes. 'How's Max?'

His heart swelled at her first words. How could he ever have doubted her?

'He's good. He's recovering and might go back to daycare next week. He's asking for you.'

'He is?'

Theo nodded, wondering where on earth he should start.

'I'm sorry,' he said simply. 'I'm sorry I doubted you, and I'm sorry I blamed you. I was wrong. I had no right to do that. And I could offer excuses—I could tell you I was panicking—I could tell you I couldn't think straight. But none of them are good enough, and I know that.'

She didn't answer. Just looked at him.

'I love you, Addy. Max loves you too. We want you in our lives. I don't care about what I heard on the phone, because I trust you. I do.'

She blinked and then licked her lips. Her voice was flat. 'I'm tired, Theo. I have an ex who has tried to ruin my life not once, but twice. Leaving me a pile of debts that weren't mine and having my house repossessed because of his actions. I came here for a fresh start. I didn't tell you any of that, because frankly I didn't think you needed to know. But he came back. With a new inspector on the case, who believed most of what came out of my ex's mouth. I was under suspicion. I went home to sort it out.'

Her violet eyes were steely.

'And all of a sudden I'm tired of not feeling in control of my own life. You walked into my apartment and treated me like crap because of a conversation you heard but didn't understand.' She put her hand on her chest. 'Can you imagine for one second how I must have felt, realising that Max had become unwell on my watch? That he needed brain surgery and I hadn't noticed or understood?'

Her voice was angry now.

'And you wouldn't let me see him! The little boy I had taken into my heart and loved as if he were my own. If things had gone wrong, I would never have got a chance to say goodbye. Can you imagine what that did to me?'

Theo raised his hands. He wanted to crawl into a hole in the ground. He was imagining if something had happened and he hadn't got a chance to say goodbye. It would have been imprinted on him for ever. He would never, ever get over something like that. And he could potentially have done that to Addy, the woman he loved. The shame was overwhelming.

'I am so, so sorry. I panicked. All I could think about was that Max was unconscious. I felt guilty because I hadn't picked him up myself. Would I have noticed anything? Probably not. Would I have done anything different from you? Probably not. But my son was sick, and I hadn't been there. Max has never been seriously ill with me before, and, the truth is, I couldn't handle it. I told you from the start I was winging it. I know nothing about being a parent, Addy. And maybe I shouldn't be. Maybe I'm not cut out for this, and Max deserves better.'

She paused, then took a breath, gesturing him over to the patchwork sofa he'd bought her. They sat down together, looking out at the skyscraper view of Dubai.

Tears were falling down her cheeks. She spoke softly but steadily. 'You are a great dad, Theo.

And you're just what Max needs. Don't doubt yourself.'

His hands were shaking. 'But look how much I messed up with you. I love you, Addy. From the bottom of my heart, I love you. *We* love you. I want us to be a family together, because I can't imagine doing this with anyone else. I wouldn't want to do this with anyone else.'

Her tears were still falling. 'But look at us, Theo. Look what happened between us. I should have told you earlier about my life back home. But I was partly ashamed. Ashamed that a man had manipulated me and committed fraud in my name. It makes me look stupid and gullible, and I didn't want that. I didn't want to tell you I'd been that person.'

'That's what affected your work?' he asked quietly.

She nodded. 'People talk. Stuart charmed people. They liked him. And when all the gossip started about fraud and money issues they looked at me differently. I could tell they were thinking I'd been involved. Can you imagine how that felt?' She shook her head, then met his gaze with her tear-stained eyes. 'It just felt like it was my own mess to clean up. I didn't want to drag you into anything. You had enough going on being a parent to Max.'

His words were gentle. 'But I could have supported you too.'

'I'm sorry,' she whispered. 'I should have trusted you. I should have told you. I'm so sorry that I didn't tell you.'

He reached over and threaded his fingers through hers. 'I'm sorry too. I'm sorry someone put you through all that. But wouldn't it be better, if something bad happens, to have someone supporting you? Someone having your back and fighting for you too?'

'Of course,' she whispered, her voice shaking.

'Then I will be,' he replied. 'From today, and for the future.' He closed his eyes for a second. She could sense he was nervous. 'We'll be there for each other.'

They interlinked their hands together and Addy leaned back into him, the warmth of her body against his. He kept talking in a low voice. 'And, if we're serious about each other, and want to be together, then should we consider Max too?' His brown eyes looked down and met hers. 'Right now, Max has only one adoptive parent. But he could have two. Then he'd be ours. Not mine.'

She let out a long, slow breath. 'My instinct is to say yes, right away. But we have a little boy's heart to consider. What if we try and we don't work?'

'We will work,' said Theo steadily. 'I'll move

heaven and earth to make us work. I can't imagine life without you.'

'And where will our future be?' she asked, looking out at the skyline.

'Wherever you want it to be.'

'I'm from Scotland. You're from France. And I know you might want to go back eventually and support your mum.'

He gave a slow nod. 'If my father's condition goes downhill, you're right, I would want to support my *maman*.' He gave her a smile. 'You have no idea how much she is going to love you.' He took a moment. 'Would you object? Would you want to stay here?'

It was Addy's turn to take a moment. It was clear she was considering things. Then she gave him a smile. 'I want to be wherever you and Max are. I can be content anywhere if I have my boys by my side.'

'You mean it?'

She nodded. 'You and Max are family to me.'

He dropped a kiss on her forehead. 'Can we really make this work?'

She gave a slow nod. 'But for Max's sake we have to take things slow. We've had a rocky few weeks. Do I want to be Max's parent? Absolutely. But let's do things at a pace that fits in with him.'

He tilted her chin up towards his and brushed a

kiss against her lips. 'I love you, Addison Bates, and I'm so glad that we found each other.'

She returned his kiss with a smile. 'I love you too, Theo Dubois. Now, let me see my boy.'

EPILOGUE

One year later

THE WEATHER IN Lyon was beautiful, and Addy couldn't wipe the smile from her face. The adoption had been finalised last month and she was now officially Max's parent.

They'd arranged their wedding in Lyon so both of Theo's parents could be there, and guests had come from Scotland and Dubai to join them.

Theo and Max were already in the hotel's gardens, standing beneath a giant arch of flowers as they waited for her. 'I have the ring,' said Max in a comic whisper to the crowd, which caused much laughter.

Her dress was a cream satin floor-length sheath, with a cowl neckline and thin diamond belt, and her bouquet was sunflowers, because yellow was now Max's favourite colour.

Her dad grinned, kissed her cheek and walked her down the garden aisle as the music started.

The last year had been so much easier than

what had come before. Stuart King had finally been jailed, and Addy had been able to give her evidence in court via video.

People at Spira had accepted them easily as a couple, and their relationship had thrived. Addy had let herself trust again, and Theo had relaxed into his role as a parent, sharing the responsibilities with someone who loved Max just as much as he did.

By the time she reached the top of the aisle Max was bouncing on his toes. 'Look at the ring,' he said proudly, opening the box and letting the diamond-set wedding band sparkle in the French sun.

She let out a little gasp—because she hadn't seen it yet. They'd skipped the engagement part and decided to move straight to the wedding.

Theo's hand slid into hers, and Max stood between them, each holding his hand as they said their wedding vows.

'I love you, Mrs Dubois,' said Theo as he slipped the ring onto her finger.

'Love you too,' she replied as she slipped his thick plain band onto his.

The celebrant lifted her arms to the crowd. 'And I now take great pleasure in pronouncing Addy and Theo as Dr and Mrs Dubois. You may kiss the bride!' she exclaimed. Theo beamed and dipped his wife backwards for a kiss.

'Me too!' shouted Max as he was lifted into their arms.

They kissed his cheeks in unison.

'To family,' Addy declared to her friends.

'To family!' they replied, and they all celebrated well into the night.

* * * * *

If you enjoyed this story,
check out these other great reads
from Scarlet Wilson

Melting Dr. Grumpy's Frozen Heart
Her Summer with the Brooding Vet
Cinderella's Kiss with the ER Doc
A Daddy for Her Twins

All available now!

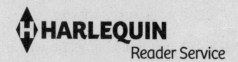

HARLEQUIN
Reader Service

Enjoyed your book?

Try the perfect subscription for Romance readers and get more great books like this delivered right to your door.

See why over 10+ million readers have tried Harlequin Reader Service.

Start with a Free Welcome Collection with free books and a gift—valued over $20.

Choose any series in print or ebook.
See website for details and order today:

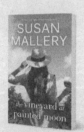
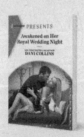
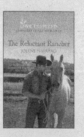
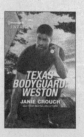

TryReaderService.com/subscriptions